IT'S A THING, IS IT?

LIVING THE LONG COVID LIFE

By

Cari Van Pieter

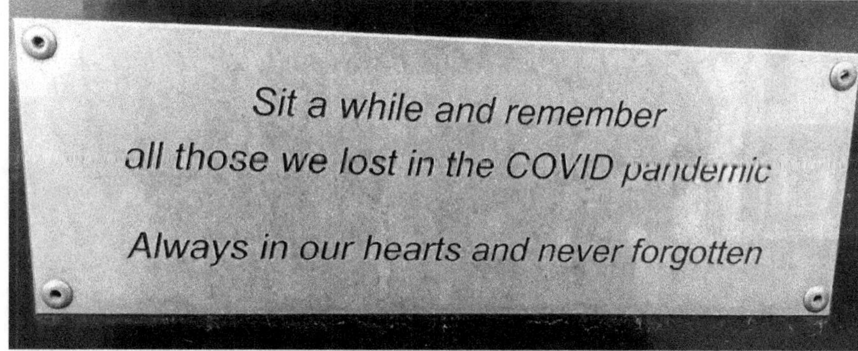

We did not lose people to death alone.
We lost and are still losing people to Long Covid.

Dedicated to all those who are suffering with Long Covid, either personally or vicariously through family or friends. You're strong, even on the weakest days. You're brave, even on the lowest days. You can hang in there, even on the days when you want to give up.

Be blessed, always.

CONTENTS

What is the point?

What is the reasoning behind this book? Well, the market may soon be flooded with works containing Long Covid advice, histories, medical specialisms. This is my take on what it is like to live with Long Covid (LC for short) long term. It's written from my point of view as a long term LC sufferer. It's not an academic work because I am neither a medical professional nor a professional academic. My aim is to reach fellow LCers and hopefully to help you feel that you are not alone and provide something you can show to the non-believers in your lives to try to help them understand. I know just how alone you can feel with LC and how no-one understands it and how you can end up feeling like a fraud, despite knowing everything you are experiencing is very real. I want you to know that there are others out here experiencing the same, who get it. You're not alone and you're not a fraud.

As I've written more and researched more, I can expand upon that. The brain fog of Long Covid means chapters of books, no matter how well written, can take forever to read and understand. What makes my book stand out? Honest answer? The bite sized chunks in the A to Z make it helpful for its audience. I can read a small section at a time without overloading my mind into brain fog status. If I'm showing it to an unwilling individual (medical or friend/family), I don't have to ask them to read 10+ pages to understand what I am trying to explain - it's a couple of paragraphs.

My less altruistic aim is to provide a catharsis for myself. I'm still trying to make sense of what has happened to me and, in writing this book, it has helped not only with my mental filing system but also has brought me a little further down the path to acceptance. I would recommend the writing process to anyone who is struggling with LC and all the "joys" it brings. It's a safe space to express whatever you feel in whatever terminology works for you. Remember, there is always a delete button for if /when you re-read your writings on another, better day!

In the beginning…

12 August 2021. Even in these new days of remembering little, that date is something I don't think I will ever be able to forget. My life changed that day because it was the day I found out that I had caught Covid-19. At first, there were the two weeks of the Delta variant infection that were pure hell to live through and survive. I was lucky not to have been hospitalised. But the legacy of Covid-19 that hit at least 65 million of us worldwide crept in silently, almost without being noticed. Two weeks after the initial infection, I wasn't recovering. Another round of antibiotics didn't shift the malaise and the confusion or restore my lost senses of taste and smell. Twelve weeks later, a walk up the hall to the front door took a good five minutes and no, I don't live in Buckingham Palace, I have a much humbler abode, where five seconds would be the usual speed. My GP, who, thank God, was on the ball with Covid and its after effects, diagnosed Long Covid.

Long Covid has taken over my life, despite my best attempts to deny it, ignore it and beat it. It is still so new that it remains elusive to concrete diagnoses through blood tests, scans etc. In turn, this promotes the disbelief similar to that experienced by those who suffer with headaches or backaches. It's invisible and can't be definitively proved so does it even exist apart from in the psyche of those claiming it? Nearly two years after GP diagnosis, I can honestly say yes, it does. The symptoms are as varied and ethereal as the disease itself and even fellow Long Covid sufferers agree that we have symptoms in common but no clear cut set of symptoms for diagnosis such as those you might see with chickenpox, for example. It's hard to lock down exactly what anyone should be looking for because Long Covid is very clever in mimicking symptoms from other illnesses, which can lead to a battery of tests with practically every hospital department, all proving negative for their speciality.

I was halfway through a talking course on Zoom with the Long Covid rehab team when I was infected again, this time with the Omicron variant of Covid-19. It was less hellish after the first few days but hold the celebration there. It added new, more painful symptoms to my already growing list, prompting a whole new set of hospital departments getting involved with a variety of new tests. It didn't take away any of the original symptoms. As for the third infection, well, that ended up in a trip to A and E for a suspected heart attack! Covid-19, the gift that keeps on giving!

Whether my life has permanently altered remains to be seen but I can say for certain that there are some changes that will never go away. Attitudinal, physical, psychological, physiological changes - they are all there to stay. Long Covid will be with me forever, even if the disease/illness eventually departs or a cure is created. It is something to be lived with. I refuse to say embraced, as I continue to loathe it as an entity for what it has done to me and others that experience it. Is it a journey? A journey implies an end is in sight but not in this case. I have had to learn that sometimes you can just look around and learn from or appreciate the getting somewhere slightly further down the line, even if you don't reach the end.

What follows is an A to Z of my thoughts, experiences, symptoms and every other jumble teased from my brain on living with Long Covid. I made it A to Z rather than a straight narrative because I can creep in and edit or add, without having to be upset about another loss of a train of thought and I know, as a Long Covid sufferer (or LCer as many of us are known), it's easier to concentrate on short pieces because the concentration's just not there for longer, more involved chapters. Some of the associations with the letters are more than a bit tenuous but please humour me! I hate a massive index with an "I know I saw that somewhere" vibe where you end up never finding what you were looking for. I stress the experiences are my own and of the people I have spoken to in person and the opinions (especially the unflattering ones) are mine alone. Where I am quoting from articles I have read or from what other LCers have told me, I hope I have made that clear and given due acknowledgement and citation.

I hope you can find what you are looking for - whether it's to identify with some of the thoughts and experiences to feel someone gets it or whether it's to try and understand those of us living the Long Covid life. If it's the former, I hope you find something that makes you feel not quite so alone. If it's the latter, thank you so much for wanting to comprehend. Good luck!

A is for…

Acceptance. Or lack thereof. One of the things that came up time and time again in the group talking sessions was the need to accept that life has changed forever with Long Covid. Or, as one therapist unsubtly put it, "The old you is dead. Accept there is a new you." 'But I don't want to,' was my first reaction. And my second. And my third. And so on through the numbers until more or less infinity. I may not have 100% liked who I was before Long Covid but I knew who I was and what I was and wasn't capable of. I could think clearly. I could function. I knew my limits and could push them without thought. Not like this new me who can't think, can't focus, can't drive far without nearly falling asleep at the wheel and has to plan the entire week ahead for a single day's activity because I have to factor in the days afterwards where I will be asleep or exhausted. This new me can't think of words, can't express herself, can't stand up for long and is in constant pain. Why should I accept it? It is unacceptable!

After a year, I noticed that I had been subconsciously making some changes. I can plan a day out, as long as I make sure the days after are free, accepting that I have the thoughts of "What if I can't make it?" and that some days just aren't going to happen. I can't multitask any more so I try to focus on one thing only. I use the words "With my Long Covid, I..." a lot. Is this acceptance? Probably not because I still hark back to what I could do pre Long Covid (or PLC as I think of it) and want desperately to be back there, mentally and physically. Is it a step on the way to acceptance? I'm going to go with yes, because I am adapting to this new life that I don't want, thereby igniting the debate of whether acceptance and adaptation are one and the same or whether one leads to the other or just simply that they are two separate entities. And that's without the whole question of resignation to my fate. Acceptance is a positive concept, an act of agreeing to something and then rolling with it, if not happily, then positively. I don't think I'm there yet but I'm trying to get there. The only thing I can be sure of is that something has to shift in my mind and attitude to make LC life a thing worth living, not just an existence. The shift has to become active acceptance, where it's a kind of "It's difficult but I can do this" vibe. The more I learn, the more I speak to other people with LC, the more research is done, the more tools I can add to the fight against LC.

Acupuncture. Whilst aimlessly googling, I found an NHS clinical study lasting for two years on the effects of acupuncture on the fatigue element of Long Covid. The aim is to see whether acupuncture can improve the symptoms of fatigue in LC sufferers. It's early days in the study yet and it will be years before the results are in. I participated in the acupuncture side and I found that it helped with cognition. Not life changing back to the way I was kind of help but a small improvement in the brain and the fatigue. Since finishing my part in the trial, I have carried on having monthly acupuncture and I still see the cognitive improvements. Is it psychological? Who cares? I will take any victory! And good luck to the doctors running the study and a big thank you for trying for us. It's great to know that we are believed, as well as that there are people out there who actually want to help.

Adapting. LC is life changing. Whatever the main symptoms for each individual are, there can be no doubt that life cannot be lived in exactly the same way as pre-Covid. Whether it's the horrors of brain fog, fatigue, breathing, pain or something else, the only way to have any quality of life for yourself and those around you is to adapt to it. Not quite an 'adapt or die' scenario but maybe an 'adapt to live' scenario instead?

I've found that out the hard way. By not listening to my body's cues and resting, I have had to deal with bigger crashes, bigger brain fog, more stammering and all the ensuing confusion. I know if I have a long, busy or stressful day, the best way I can try to mitigate the inevitable fatigue is to try to plan two or three days afterwards of quiet, low brain and low physical activity. It's annoying and not always easy to do and exceptionally frustrating but by adapting the lifestyle to the illness, I've managed to have a better quality of the new life I am stuck with.

Ambition vs ability. It's something I say quite a lot now: "My ambition has exceeded my ability." I still plan things or want to do things the old way, be that a holiday (remember those?!) or a daily task. That's when the plan or what I plan based on old patterns goes horribly wrong. I can't function at those levels any more, even if those levels were not particularly high functioning or achieving. I have to consider the LC effect upon daily life, including absentia from that life, in every plan. When I don't - I'm not even going to say 'if' here - I fail in the plan somewhere. For example, when we used to have a holiday, a day was not complete without having visited a minimum of two places of interest. Now, if I try and keep functioning at that level, I may succeed on the first day and I may even achieve it on the second. By the third, however, I can barely move and by the fourth, I am sleeping and/or on painkillers for the rest of the week.

This tells me I need to adapt my ambition of what I think I can achieve to match it with my ability. LC is sneaky. Very sneaky. I can do one day (if I'm lucky) at my old functioning levels and sometimes, I don't seem to have any detrimental side effects the following day. Invariably, this leads to me becoming overambitious on the second day, leading to the inevitable crash on day three. And four. And five. You get the picture. If I do one day okay, sometimes the next day is a day of crashing, sleeping and pain. In other words, I have no way of predicting which way LC will sneak up on me. All I can guarantee is that I get it wrong more times than I get it right and my ambition always exceeds my ability, leading to regular frustration and disappointment for me and for those around me. And lots of ugly crying. It happens. It goes back to acceptance. If I can become more accepting of my LC, my ambition and ability may balance out more.

Anger. When you have had a life taken away by Long Covid and all its minions, you get very angry. I know this. I am angry with LC, angry with myself for not being able to 'get over it', angry with the medical profession who dismiss my needs out of hand, angry with God for letting me carry on living this half life, angry with relatives who just won't understand and roll their eyes every time LC is mentioned - the list goes on forever. Anger can take over but on some days, it's just too much effort to even get angry, which makes the rage levels get worse.

It's not fair to take it out on those around me but it happens. Anger can be all pervading, all consuming and blind you to the need to adapt and accept. Pre LC life is over. Some people have been lucky enough for LC to go away and leave them relatively unscathed but for the longer term LC sufferer, there is no end in sight. New symptoms appear on a regular basis and take over. Anger at it all never leaves. Anger at the person who gave you Covid in the first place. Anger at the enforced changes in life. Anger at life and ability being dramatically changed by an external force and with no personal input into it. LC is cruel.

The only thing to do with the anger is to try to channel it to make it manageable before every relationship in your life is destroyed. I am writing this guide as a way of expressing what is going on in my head and it does help with the anger management, as it is quite a cathartic experience. Don't get me wrong, I get flares of anger over ridiculously small things as well as large ones. It's not unreasonable in my mind that it happens because it can also be a catalyst in forcing me out to look for help and forcing me to try things that are well out of my comfort zone to try and recover. The anger that can trigger an "I'll show you" response to LC. Anger has a place and is an entirely reasonable thing to be feeling but it needs to be channelled before it gets destructive.

Anxiety. Like the anger levels, anxiety can reach a new high. From the obvious and perhaps simplistic thoughts of "Will I never get better?", through the concerns that Long Covid will alienate those around you, right up to the disaster planning thoughts of "LC will end up killing me," anxiety lurks around every corner. I'd like to say that the anxiety fades the longer LC goes on but it doesn't. Even if one particular set of concerns is resolved, others pop up to take its place. It seems more heightened and internalised than pre-LC anxiety levels, maybe because there is so much uncertainty about (a) the actual longevity of LC, (b) what its permanent effects on the mind and body are and (c) the fact that it is an invisible illness.

Anxiety is the uncomfortable relative that comes with LC, co-dependant on one another for survival. It can be crippling, debilitating and affects everyone and everything. Panic attacks caused by anxiety have become a more regular feature of my everyday life. I have ended up in Accident and Emergency with what was thought to be a heart attack but was actually a severe panic attack coupled with or even triggered by costochondritis and another Covid 19 infection. That time meant I couldn't go on holiday abroad as they couldn't rule out heart issues, so severe was the effect on my heart and blood pressure of both the Covid 19 and the anxiety. As it was a few hours before my flight and I was still in A and E, that holiday was just not going to happen. That's where guilt takes over because it's not just me that gets affected by the results of anxiety, it's my family and friends too.

I tried CBT to help reduce the spiking levels of anxiety that are now dominating my life but was discharged by the therapist because I wasn't ready for it, apparently. (No, I still don't get it!) That sent me back to square one with both anxiety and depression because I felt that there's just no help out there for me. Yes, I know it's ultimately down to me to beat this or at least take it down to manageable levels but a bit of help and support would boost my confidence no end. Anxiety just takes over everything and even going to the corner shop is a long internal debate, involving palpitations, cold sweats and other physical manifestations and that's without the fatigue factor.

LC has intensified anxiety in me and forced it to the front of every plan I make, every action I take. It has made me question myself and my abilities. When booking holidays, my ability is nowhere near as competent as my ambition and the panic sets in as my anxiety levels spike. What if I get exhausted with LC and can't follow the itinerary and get stuck? What if I become ill and need to get home? Too many thoughts clog up my reasoning and the waves of terror overcome any desire I have to do anything, meaning I am stuck at home, shivering with guilt and terror. But I'm not ready for any treatment from a psychologist yet, they say. What's the answer? Nothing I can think of.

Anxiety also shoulders the blame for when any test results ordered by GPs, hospital consultants etc show up negative. "Well, it must be anxiety triggering … fill in the blank with your symptoms here…" I am in no position to deny that sometimes it is all down to anxiety and nothing terrible is going on physiologically. However, absence of positive results is all too often laid at anxiety's door when it really isn't the case. As someone who suffers with anxiety, believe it or not, I can tell the difference most of the time. Anxiety is the whipping boy of medical ignorance and it is concerning that important biological changes are being missed because everything is being swept away under the banner of anxiety.

Anxiety exists big time. Anxiety can be crippling and can increase to life changing levels. LC has definitely increased my anxiety levels about every aspect of my life, as well as my concerns for those around me. Everything has magnified to ridiculous disproportion. But not all the LC symptoms are anxiety based and shouldn't be judged to be so just because there are no positive results in standard tests. It's amazing how much is written off as anxiety just because test results show negative. The questionnaires I get given to fill in are the anxiety and depression ones - not an unreasonable thing - but there seems to be little thought given to LC having invisible symptoms. Invisible to standard test results, that is. I know what has changed and is changing and it is very annoying as well as frustrating to have it written off as the anxiety of a postmenopausal woman almost every time.

Attention span. This book seems to have taken forever to write because my attention span rivals that of the much maligned goldfish. A few words into a sentence and I feel my thoughts drifting off to something else, losing not only the train of thought but also the ability to form meaningful words. If someone is talking to me, I find after a few sentences, I'm off with the fairies (or goldfish!) and not able to focus on what is being said to me. Annoying for friends and family but concerning for me when it's a medical person giving me information, instructions or advice.

I used to be able to concentrate for hours on end on a topic or conversation. Now, it's more like two minutes and that's on a good day. That's another reason why this book is written the way it is. For me as the author, I'd be forever losing my train of thought and coming back to it not having a clue what I was writing about. By slicing it into 26 sections with numerous subsections, I've been able - finally - to get it all down on paper. The number of extra subsections that could have existed in the book but don't are legion because I've thought of a heading, continued with what I'm typing and then lost the headings, remembering only that I'd thought of them. I lost 2 just in this last paragraph! In case anyone reading also has this attention span loss, hopefully, the short sections and subsections will make it easier for you to dive in and out without feeling the pressure of having to finish a chapter or so many pages at a time.

Driving seems ok until I have to remember where I am going! Numerous times, I've pulled over because I've forgotten which turn the Satnav told me to take or I've seen a sign pointing to somewhere interesting and I've thought about that and forgotten the original destination. No retention and no attention span - a fun place not to be!

<u>B is for…</u>

Balance. The number of LCers who say their balance has gone wonky since having Covid has surprised me. I had assumed my inability to stand on one leg before crashing Godzilla-like to the floor was an age thing or a me thing. I've never had brilliant balance but it used to be so much better prior to Covid. Now, I wobble if a toe leaves the floor. There doesn't seem to be any conclusive evidence that Covid is to blame but the number of LCers that report their ability to balance has deteriorated makes me wonder. One of the lovely physios involved with the LC rehab group has shown us some exercises to try and improve it and they do help, as long as you manage to keep on doing them. The problem isn't solved but it is helped. I'm not sure it is an LC thing but I thought I would include it here because in a group of 8 LCers, 5 are having balance problems so it could be considered to be a symptom or effect of it. I reiterate that I have no medical qualifications and my observations are just that - observations. Food for thought, maybe?

Baseline. "Find your baseline. Establish a baseline," was a constant piece of advice from the Zoom rehab team. A fine principle but very difficult without one to one help to understand it all and even more difficult when your life doesn't follow the standard 9 to 5 routine. *The Long Covid self-help guide* explains the ideas far better than I can but essentially, finding a baseline is all about managing the crashing fatigue that LC brings. Not tiredness, fatigue.

A baseline is about what you can manage to do in a day without triggering fatigue and all its friends. It's a kind of basis for living. If I go way over my baseline, I know I'll be paying in terms of LC flare up for days, sometimes even weeks, depending how badly I've gone over my limit. If I manage to stay on the baseline, doing what I can do, then I can just about manage to get through a day. It is a one day at a time thing.

It's also a bit like a budget, in that you can plan ahead for a big spend. If I know I'm going out, then I make sure I have a quiet few days before and after. Does that avoid the crash? It's not that kind of budget, where saving up equals a lot to spend. It's more like knowing when your big spend is coming and knowing, as a result, you'll be living on bread and water for a while afterwards. Planning is key and to be able to plan, you can try and work out when the crash will come after a major spend.

That being said, the whole idea of a baseline is to avoid this kind of boom and bust. The books and the clinicians will give a full on account of how to plan ahead so that the crash 'rarely' happens. I'm talking about a practical, more realistic life. Kids, parents, partners, friends, work, pets and everything in between can get in the way of the smooth baseline thinking. I'm not advocating a boom and bust lifestyle because that would be incredibly destructive and unhelpful in managing LC. I'm suggesting you work out the baseline which works best for you so you know you can make it through a day, then be realistic if you know you're going to have to go over that baseline by trying to lie low afterwards. I have found that this type of planning ahead helps me mentally before the big spend up because I don't feel a pressure to keep going afterwards. If it's a continual spend that has to happen, the only thing I can suggest is looking for the downtime around the sides of it and taking time out of the situations wherever possible. I've found hiding in the toilet for 10 minutes can help!

Blood pressure. Another little by-product of Covid that has hit me is a steep rise in my blood pressure. According to Ged Medinger's long term effects of Covid chart in *The Long Covid Handbook*, it affects 1% of other LCers too. Trying to convince the GP that I need something sorting has taken more than a year but, at last, I seem to be on the endless cycle of trying to find the right blood pressure tablet for me. The biggest problem I'm having with the blood pressure pills (apart from the seemingly inescapable swelling and itchiness that come hand in hand with each type) is that they all seem to trigger my LC fatigue. I'm hoping it's a case of persevering until I get to the right one and that the combined patience of me and my GP lasts that long! Just when I seemed to have established a vague baseline for everyday life, one 2.5mg pill seems to have sent me back down the fatigue ladder, with more hours spent in bed than upright.

After four different types of blood pressure pill and a very narrow escape from being in Intensive Care due to a severe allergic reaction to one of those pills, I seem to have found 'the one'! Even then, at the smallest possible 1.25mg dose as part of a slow release mechanism, it was too much for me. LC has made me hypersensitive to many drugs, blood pressure ones being some of them. I wasn't having the terrible side effects but I spent 18 hours a day asleep. A review with the GP showed that even that dose, combined with LC's hypersensitivity, had sent my blood pressure into the 'too low' bracket. Halving the pill and taking it at night (i.e. going against all the manufacturer's guidelines) seems to have worked. It's like getting a sleeping pill into the bargain. The chemist wasn't happy to release my medication because the pills are meant to be taken in the morning and whole, not split into two, because of the whole slow release thing. Once I explained, because she was an LC sufferer too, she understood and I can now get my meds with no question. It's under 6 monthly review with the GP but for now, fingers crossed, my blood pressure is under control. Blood pressure - yet another thing LC messes with!

Blood tests. Oh, there have been so many blood tests since I first had Covid. The only useful thing they have shown is what isn't wrong! Is LC particularly sneaky and hides itself? Or is it there with all horns blaring and waving but the markers to identify it as LC just haven't been found yet? Hopefully, one day they will be but in the meantime, I just smile and nod when I'm asked to go for a blood test and smile and nod again when I'm told there's nothing showing up. Maybe the medics will find some blood markers and we can be official LC sufferers. If it's too sneaky for them, let's just hope there's another type of test coming soon that can yell, "Aha! Gotcha!" and find LC lurking in the bloodstream.

On 7 February 2023, The Times reported that an American company was offering (for a price, naturally!) blood tests to confirm the presence of Long Covid. Should the result be positive, they then offer drugs to break the "spike protein" of Covid-19, thereby offering a cure of sorts. It's up to the individual to decide to go down this route or not. My personal opinion is that the long arm of LC is too far reaching to be cured by drugs being used off-label. In my opinion, all the consequences of LC are still coming to light and I don't want to risk what health I currently have by chasing down a rabbit hole that makes it worse. Having said that, the fact that there is now some kind of blood test out there offers a glimmer of hope that eventually a mainstream blood test will be developed to prove LC exists, not only to the sufferers and their families but to the doubters within the medical profession.

Brain Fog. For me, this is the worst part of Long Covid. Brain fog is where nothing makes sense any more - you can't think coherently; you can't string a sentence together because you can't remember words, names, day to day things; you can't understand what someone is saying to you because you hear the words but the brain doesn't put them into anything you can understand; you have no ability to concentrate and anything over a minute long is impossible to grasp before the brain shuts down; you get overwhelmed if more than one person is talking because it's overloading the senses and the brain won't file it for you; you're standing like a sheep waiting to be told what to do because you just can't remember what you are meant to be doing; you need to write everything down from every conversation with everyone because you won't remember anything that was said in five minutes' time.

It's crying with frustration; it's feeling terror that dementia has come calling because so many of the brain fog symptoms are similar to dementia symptoms; it's lowering the IQ; it's memory loss; it's feeling a huge sense of loss for the brain that you once had; it's mourning the person you were. It's a nightmare that I just can't seem to wake up from and have no idea how to.

I've been in a public toilet with a slide across bolt and had to phone my daughter who was waiting outside to ask her how to get out because I just couldn't understand how the bolt works. I've been standing by a hospital door hoping someone will come through it because I couldn't figure out how to make it open. I've been thrown out of a sandwich shop because they thought I was drunk or on drugs because I just couldn't get the words 'meal deal' into my head and out of my mouth and was coming out with things like, "I want the drink but not the drink and the sandwich but not the sandwich," which probably justified their believing I was not sober. A fellow LCer has literally run out of a restaurant in floods of tears and stood dry heaving by the side of the road because a group of friends she was with had a conversation which she just couldn't follow and she had ended up getting overwhelmed by the words, lights and situation.

On a day to day basis, I know I have about half an hour of reasonable brain activity, which is when I try to get things like bills paid, appointments made etc. After that, it's hit and miss, with the greater part of the day consisting of me starting a job and forgetting that I am doing it. For example, things like the washing gets loaded into the machine but I don't remember to turn it on so it sits there all day until someone else notices it isn't even wet. It's like living a weird quarter life where it's a rush to fit in the essentials before the fog descends again and there's no avoiding it. For someone who used to be quite bright, brain fog is a living nightmare and by far the most devastating part of LC for me.

It is also heartbreaking when you can tell that those close to you think you are making it up for attention, are being lazy or for some other reason. The impatience, the eye rolls, the sighs, the 'never minds' all add up and grind the frustration gears up a notch. The not being able to find a word and either grunting and gesturing or using a completely incorrect word isn't easily understood unless you have that brain fog that just removes everything you know from your grasp. I've tried the mind boosting apps on my phone, meditation to clear away the noise, memory exercises and more but the fog continues to come down. It really is devastating.

Breathing. Breathing is natural and you don't have to think about it, right? Up until LC struck, I would have agreed. I was lucky not to have been hospitalised with Covid so I can't talk about the effects of Covid upon breathing where it's so tough that a ventilator has to be used to keep you going. But I can talk about the fact that I sometimes gasp for breath, not through lack of fitness but through inability to fill my lungs properly. A lady in my LC group commented that she had to have physiotherapy to teach her how to breathe properly again.

Apparently, Covid can affect the pattern of breathing so that only the top part of the lung is used, making the lower part almost redundant. That leads to less air/oxygen being taken in with each breath and so a drop in oxygen saturation levels. A prolonged drop in these levels can cause so many more difficulties. I started measuring my saturation levels once I discovered this, confident that my readings would still be their pre-Covid 99-100% levels. I was shocked to find a daily average of 95%, with lows of 92% being far too regular. 92% is great for a GCSE result but for oxygen saturation, the NHS warn that it may be a sign of hypoxia (where oxygen isn't reaching the body's tissues properly).

I realised that the speed of my breathing was increasing to try and grab that oxygen out of the air but actually achieving nothing other than making me more breathless and inducing a feeling of panic. I went back to the advice from my fellow LCer and investigated breathing techniques while waiting for the physio appointment. It turns out there are a plethora of techniques for breathing to use the bottom part of the lungs, as well as increasing capacity and endurance. A quick Google or YouTube search will show you the variety of techniques available, along with easy to follow demonstrations. I have been trying some of them and my oxygen saturation level has increased to an average of 96%, while the feeling of panic at not being able to catch my breath properly is receding.

Breathlessness. Different from not being able to catch your breath. It's a constant state of not being able to pull in enough air. It can be terrifying because you breathe faster and faster trying to drag oxygen into your lungs, creating a feeling of panic. This leads to a racing heart and blind terror. I am fortunate in that I was only affected by the breathlessness whilst I had Covid but that was enough for me! I know of fellow LCers who have this problem every day, more than three years after their initial Covid infection. Salbutamol (a drug for asthma) is often prescribed but does not always have the desired effect. It's important to get to see a pulmonary specialist as soon as possible, even if the only achievement is to have heart problems ruled out. I say a pulmonary specialist rather than a cardiac one because heart problems can present as breathlessness and a pulmonary consultant specialises in lung disorders.

In short, I don't have much experience with the breathlessness so I'm not going to make stuff up just to fill space. If there is any concern, use an oximeter and get medical help as soon as you can.

C is for...

Cards. Watching the *Joker* film, the part where Arthur Fleck hands over a card explaining his uncontrollable laughter made me think, "This is what I need." I've been asked to leave shops because they thought I was drunk or on drugs because I couldn't put the words together to ask for what I wanted to purchase and I certainly didn't have the words to explain LC. Trying to get people to give me those precious minutes to gather my thoughts and utter some words is very hard sometimes. I saw Arthur Fleck's card as a moment of genius that could explain everything that I couldn't. Not everything with LC can be covered on a credit card sized explanation but it should be possible to get enough on one to succinctly say, "Give me time, I'll get there."

My idea was solid but I put nothing into practise due to my own inertia and lack of resources. Then, when idling browsing the internet one day, I found these cards actually exist for LCers as part of the worldwide Hidden Disabilities sunflower scheme (www.hiddendisabilitiesstore.com). To know these cards exist and are available for LCers to purchase is an amazing step forward for me and other LCers that I have told about them. The cards read, "Please be patient with me. I have fatigue and can have trouble breathing so may need to rest. I can become confused and may need more time to communicate with you." And that really does the job in giving me the time and space to be able to do, think or say whatever I need to. It is available internationally too!

I can honestly say that having the card, even when I'm not using it on a lanyard around my neck, has restored some of my confidence when out and about. Knowing an explanation is easily available in my handbag to be shown when needed has made me relax more and feel I can go into places that I had extreme anxiety about visiting after being thrown out of shops. A paramedic friend suggested to me that I should wear it if on a longer journey in the car or on a coach so if there is an accident, any potential rescuers can see that I may have communication difficulties that may not be injury related and give me the time I may need to respond. In short, for me, these cards, whilst labelling me, have restored a lot of confidence in my ability to interact with others outside the home.

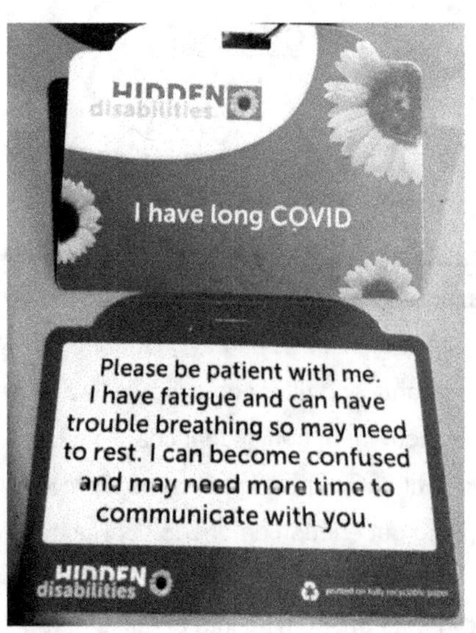

Chilblains. Having treatment on my unrelated to LC ingrowing toenail, the podiatrist commented that my toes were covered in chilblains. I knew this was the case following a particularly grim winter but it is unusual for me to have had them go on for seven months. I mentioned this to her, saying I had had the odd chilblain appear randomly over the years but never on every toe at the same time and for such a long period of time. We talked about Covid Toe but, although there are similarities in appearance, I only had the one Covid Toe. The rest of the mess was an outbreak of chilblains.

I commented that I had never had so many chilblains but, since my first Covid infection, it was turning into an annual event for me, with each year's outbreak being worse and more long-lived than the previous year. 2022 into 2023 had recurrence after recurrence of chilblains, ensuring a very painful walk and almost unnoticeable recovery. Changing my slip on shoes to laced ones and wearing heated insoles with two thinner pairs of socks had little effect, which was as puzzling to the podiatrist as it was to me. As soon as I mentioned Covid/LC, she looked at me as if a lightbulb had gone on. "We've had to treat so many more chilblains since Covid started," were her startled words to me.

I can't say for sure that chilblains are another effect of LC or even Covid itself but to hear from a podiatrist that the outbreaks are more widespread than in the pre-Covid period does make me wonder why. It could be a side-effect of lockdown, of course, a bit like the whole immune system decline but there could be something in it, like the whole balance issue. I'm not qualified to say but again am including it as something that has changed in me and seemingly in other people since the brush with Covid.

Codes. According to NHS ENgland's website, "SNOMED CT is a structured clinical vocabulary for use in an electronic health record. It is the most comprehensive and precise clinical health terminology product in the world, forming an integral part of the electronic care record. It represents care information in a clear, consistent, and comprehensive manner." There is a code for every condition, referral, signposting, assessment and outcome measure. No, I didn't know that either! These codes should be attached to your electronic NHS record and there's a whole wave of them dedicated to Covid-19 and Post Covid Syndrome (Long Covid).

"1325161000000102 Post-COVID-19 syndrome (disorder)" is the one that every LC sufferer should have in their records. It may even help with the "I have Long Covid" speech at the start of any hospital appointment as it will be there ready for the practitioner to read, rather than waiting for the LCer to explain why they are the way they are. I will certainly be chatting to my GP on my next visit, asking if the code is attached to me and requesting that it is. What is surprising is how many codes there are, showing all assessment tools, signposts and referrals that many, like me, will have never had access to. Maybe it's a lack of medical professional awareness of how far-reaching LC can be?

Conspiracy theory. There are so many conspiracy theories out there on the origins of Covid and LC and I'm not getting into them here. David Gardner does a great job of looking at many of them in his book *Covid 19: The Conspiracy Theories* if you'd like to read more. There are conspiracy theories about LC too circulating in social media, like it being a tool for controlling people they couldn't kill; control of women (hello, what about the men who have it?!); a version of a new more deadly virus sitting dormant in LCers until some kind of D-Day and so on and so on. There will always be conspiracy theories about pretty much anything so it shouldn't be a surprise that LC gets its face in there. Honestly, I'm not that concerned about why and am more bothered about them finding a cure than pointing fingers. The downside of all the conspiracy gossip is that often it detracts from finding the reasoning or cure behind the event. If there was a bit less social media frenzy on conspiracy theories behind Covid and LC and a lot more social media demand for finding a cure for both, we could all potentially be in a better situation faster.

Cost-benefit. It seems like every day is a constant planning phase of my life. If I know I have a big energy expense coming up, I have to weigh up whether the benefit of doing whatever I need/want to do outweighs what it will cost me in terms of fatigue, brain fog, depression and so on. Sometimes, it's an easy decision like when I had to take my father to the cancer hospital and stay with him for test results, which resulted in the following day where I had to ask my daughter how to turn the hoover off because I just hadn't a clue how to make it stop, followed by a couple of hours in bed, exhausted. The benefit of that decision outweighed the personal cost, in my opinion.

Sometimes, it's not so easy because LC is very unpredictable or it doesn't seem like there is a big decision to be made. I hadn't thought that going out for a coffee with a friend would leave me in a completely brain fogged state, unable to do anything or understand what was going on around me for the rest of the day. Did that cost outweigh the benefit of seeing my friend? I'd like to say no but it's an awful feeling letting someone down so the jury is still out on that one. I couldn't have predicted that was how my LC would get to me that time so hadn't done a 'correct' calculation on the cost-benefit scale. LC is sneaky like that.

Learning from that experience, I try to look at the week ahead, knowing what plans have been made and weigh up what is worth the benefit and what is just not worth the cost of doing. It's neither a proactive nor reactive way of thinking because it falls between both and is neither acceptance nor resignation. It comes under adaptation more than any other type of thought process. It's not something I enjoy doing; it's not even 90% reliable but it's a way of getting through the days with as clear a conscience as possible for those around me, as well as making LC life a tad more liveable.

Cough. The cough is a huge part of Covid 19 and all the paperwork associated with it. 'Do you have a new, persistent cough?' appears on documents from hospitals, dentists, theatres - you name it. Something I have noticed since my LC started is the dry cough that seems to be a permanent feature now in my life. It's not a 24/7 thing that never ceases but I guarantee that, at some point every day, I will be coughing for a short while. My chest always feels congested now and my guess is that the cough is trying to clear that congestion. It's been suggested to me that it's just a habit. I'm not sure I agree because it isn't something I feel I can control. Chest feeling full and heavy equals need to cough. It's not even an annoyance really; it's just there all the time. When the question is 'new, persistent cough', it's an easy 'no' response. When the question is 'continuous cough', the answer is not so simple. A bit like the 'have you lost your sense of taste and smell?' question, the answer is 'no more than usual,' which leads to a whole host of other queries. Tough one to call when you combine the cough with the lung patches left by LC. I don't really have an answer for whether or not it's a habit or LC damage but it's a new part of me.

Covid Toe. Something else that comes under the "It's a thing, is it?" and mimicry talents of Covid. Covid Toe is when the toe gets all red and swollen as if you have chilblains, complete with a little bag of pus as if it is infected. And it hurts a lot. It is neither chilblains nor infection in that sense. It is another gift from Covid. The purple scabs afterwards are a delight to behold too. If you're really lucky, like me, nine out of your ten toes will have Covid Toe. It's a beast, really, because even after it clears up having had hydrocortisone creams, antifungals and antibiotics thrown at it, I've been left with some strange looking rows of scars on the toes. When winter comes, despite layers of socks, heated insoles, fastening shoes as opposed to slip ons, the chilblains from hell then start on the rows of scars, making them all red and swollen again. Mercifully, no more bags of pus though. It's hard to know now whether I have recurring Covid Toe with my LC or whether it has just weakened the skin and decreased the immune system so much that I have year long chilblains. And an odd, hobbling walk due to my painful toes!

Crashing. You can't move to put one foot in front of another. You can't speak, just stammer the first letter of what you want to say. You can't think. No coherent thoughts run through your head. If someone speaks to you, it's just a series of incomprehensible sounds that just wash over you. That's a Long Covid crash. The only thing to do is go to bed and stay there until it passes, which is inconvenient at best and soul destroying at worst. Overdoing it in whatever way - physical, mental, emotional - can bring on a crash.

Clues that it is coming are there when the ultra fatigue kicks in, the hoarseness and the no sense of words flood the brain. I try to go for that lie down before it hits the real crash because then I may only be out of it for a day. Sometimes it works, sometimes it doesn't. On days where I know I have to overdo it, I keep the following days free in case of a crash. Obviously, the thing to do is not overdo it and not bring on a crash but real life doesn't always work that way!

Sometimes, a crash just happens without warning. I was in the car park at Tesco, having done the week's shop and suddenly, I just couldn't move. Literally, I was frozen to the spot. Luckily, I was with my husband and I was able to grunt out, "Car," and he brought the car round, bent me into a sitting position and drove home, where I made it as far as the hall before just sitting in a heap on the floor. Those crashes are the worst because you can't plan for them and you can end up in a difficult situation if there's no one out there with you.

It could seem that the only thing to do then with LC is stay at home in fear of the next crash. Again, that goes back to the choice between living and existing. Some days, existing is the only option but to actually live with LC, crashing and all the components of surviving each crash, comes down to planning and accepting that it's just going to be that way until there's either a cure or it goes away. Maybe forever, then.

Cures. It was inevitable that cures for LC began to be touted around the internet, in the newspapers and so on. On 21 May 2023, the *Mail Online* shared exciting news that for a mere (!) £10,000 a week, LC sufferers could go to a clinic in Spain for an amazing treatment that could potentially cure them. Hmm, well, I can't expand on the science or theories behind it but 10k a week sounds a very good cure for the therapists' bank balances! Let's face it, most of us LCers don't have that kind of cash to splash, even if the hope it offers is huge.

Hope is a big thing for me because I desperately want to get well. There are so many quacks out there offering this, that and the other as a potential LC cure, desperation and vain hope could easily drain 10k from your pocket in dribs and drabs, without a fancy clinic stay to show for it. Throughout history, as soon as there is an illness or a problem, a plethora of 'cures' become available for the gullible, the despairing and the hopeful. LC is the latest in that very long line and its 205 known symptoms make it easy for a vast range of treatments to flood the market. Some of the quack cures may do far more harm than good and Caveat Emptor certainly applies big time! I live in hope that a cure will one day be found but am realistic enough to know it may not be in my lifetime. I am happy to try anything suggested that doesn't have the potential to harm me (or my wallet!) because you never know and something may genuinely help but clutching at 10k a pop straws is not the way forward for me.

<u>D is for...</u>

Denial. Denial takes many forms. The most familiar is the denial by the medics that LC is a thing and that if your blood tests, X-Rays, CT scans, MRIs etc show up as normal, then there is nothing wrong with you so it must be anxiety. Denial can come from those closest to you as well. The hardest is complete denial that there is anything wrong apart from hypochondria and attention seeking. Even initial sympathy can turn to the "Aren't you better yet?" type of denial that LC is a long term prospect or even permanent. Expectation that you will be exactly the same as before the initial Covid infection is high, followed by disappointment and annoyance that you are not. It's another form of denial.

It's easy to be judgmental about others but self denial can be the biggest problem of all. Acceptance, adaptation and even motivation can only occur properly once denial has been defeated. Self denial can again take many forms. Mentally, I have been through the "I will beat this," stage, through the "It's not real," stage, through the "I will carry on like I did before," stage, through the "I'm just being pathetic," stage and through the "I can't let everyone down," stage. All of these stages are denying that LC is here to stay and has changed my life and my abilities. And they keep coming back too in an endless loop. When I say I have been through these stages, I guess what I really mean is I'm constantly going through these stages in turn.

Self denial can be defeated but it's a war, not just one battle. Like LC, it's always lurking there. Every time when I deliberately don't listen to my body's cues; every time when I deliberately push myself past where I know my body and mind can go now, the denial that LC is there is winning the war. Sometimes it's a conscious denial and sometimes it is not. What I know for sure is that if I deny my LC and push past the boundaries, I pay for it days afterwards with the fatigue kicking in and making normal - even the new normal - functioning impossible.

Pushing the mental side is actually harder because my brain just literally shuts down when it reaches tolerance point. Because of the continual brain fog, it's hard to say whether I pay for overdoing it on the days that follow. I think it seems harder to concentrate, to understand and to function cognitively but it's not as clear cut as the physical overreaching. Whatever the truth, denial of LC does me no favours, so I need to move to acceptance, no matter how reluctantly, in order to live to what is the best possible ability.

Depression. Feeling low is to depression what tiredness is to fatigue - it's what people think they understand about the word but is a million miles away from the truth, which is far darker, more gnarly and 100% more terrifying. I suffered from depression long before Covid, for over 30 years now. It creeps up on you when your body is low, not just your mind. Gez Medinger makes it clear in *The Long Covid Handbook* that LC symptoms are nothing to do with pre-existing depression or anxiety, as many GPs are keen to attribute it to. LC and depression are different animals and should be treated as such.

Prior to my first Covid infection, I was in a pretty good headspace by my standards. I was looking after my adored granddaughter, awaiting the birth of my grandson and life was sweet. Covid struck, affecting us all - me, my pregnant daughter and my grandbaby. Each day was a struggle to breathe, to move and to stay alive. As those symptoms receded, for the others at least, the depression came bounding back like an evil hound, biting back into my psyche and taking over again.

Every day since has been yet another battle with depression. The longevity and seemingly eternal life of LC has added more and more to the feeling of never ending hopelessness. Every emotional factor that comprises LC seems to add fuel to the fires of depression - the fatigue, the anger, the grief, the guilt - the list is seemingly endless. I can't begin to claim that depression is a symptom of LC but it can come bounding up to play a result of it. Some of the antidepressants prescribed make the fatigue worse, which leads to feeling more depressed about LC, which contributes to the never-ending cycle of depression. The key to that is to keep working with a GP to find the right antidepressants for you and your body (and for the financially conscious, if you pay for prescriptions, invest in the annual pre-payment certificate! I estimate it has saved me over £100 in the first three months since purchase.)

Antidepressants aren't always the solution and I neither advocate nor don't advocate their use. It's an individual choice but be aware that if you go down that route, you don't have to stick to the first drug prescribed. If it's not helping or making it all worse, get it changed or stopped. Don't do what I did and stop taking a very high dose overnight. Believe me, it took me four months to be free of some horrific side-effects that, if I'd reduced them and come off with my GP's supervision, I would not have experienced in such an extreme way. I now don't touch them, despite the tiny voice that talks sense into me telling me I may need to again!

Depression is sneaky. You have a good day and think you're okay, only to be caught out a few days later with some exceptionally bad days/weeks/months. It's very like LC in that respect. There are a lot of books, therapies, websites and so on about depression so I'm not going to carry on about it. I just wanted to make that nod to LC and depression because it is yet another one of those LC symptoms out there. As to depression itself, there is no answer other than keep talking to the GP or consultant, take up talking therapies (or at least join a waiting list!) and continue trying to keep your head above water. The waiting list for help is endless and is to be endured. Depression, like LC, is an endurance event. I have no good advice to offer other than keep asking for help, keep trying and make the most of any good moments that come your way.

Disability. *The New York Times* suggested that LC could be "one of the largest mass disabling events in modern history," on 17 March 2021. (https://www.nytimes.com/2021/03/17/opinion/long-covid.html) The numbers of LC sufferers have grown to well over 65 million people worldwide and the numbers seem sure to increase with no concrete cause or cure on the horizon. But is LC a disability? It's a huge question that can probably only be best tackled in a book of its own with arguments back and forth on both sides but it's still worth a brief few lines here as a nod to the enormity of the problem.

There is no doubt among LC sufferers that it is disabling, taking away 'normality' and creating problems. But is that a disability? Under the UK's Equality Act 2010, a disability is a "physical or mental impairment that has a 'substantial' and 'long-term' negative effect on your ability to do normal daily activities". Long term is defined as over 12 months. According to this definition, then, all of us with LC who are racking up the anniversaries of initial infection can be classed as disabled. It can be argued that disabling is not the same as disabled. It's a label that some would shy away from, others would embrace and a few would exploit. There's no right or wrong answer and I feel it's up to the individual whether they chose to think of themself as disabled by LC and whether having LC for more than a year is a disability.

Dizziness. After my second bout of Covid, I noticed an increase in dizziness, real room spinning dizziness. It didn't seem to matter whether I was going from sitting to standing, walking around or even lying in bed. I'd be reaching for something to hold on to because it felt as though I was about to fall. It was different to the balance thing where I couldn't balance properly and felt a bit wonky. I asked my GP to check for signs of an ear infection and there were none. Talking to other LCers, it seems that dizziness is quite a thing amongst us. Some people have it very badly and develop PoTS (postural orthostatic tachycardia syndrome) where the heart rate suddenly increases to ridiculously fast levels, causing dizziness on standing or sitting up. I'm lucky to have avoided that so far but some LCers in my group have been very badly affected by it.

I have been "lucky" with the dizziness and the symptoms have receded over the months. I have the occasional dizzy spell but that could be down to blood pressure or not eating enough now. The rehab physios gave me some exercises to do to help and they really seem to have done the trick, along with staying well hydrated. They are the same as the balance ones, so I have killed two birds with one stone. Having read about dizziness, it seems that it can be a symptom of a viral infection so it would fit with the timeline of turning up during and after Covid.

<u>E is for...</u>

Energy bank. I've seen LC fatigue compared to a battery, a bank balance and many other things. Essentially, it's a tool for helping those without LC understand that a good sleep won't solve the energy crisis. Not all energy expended is physical but all types add up to a huge expenditure that is incredibly difficult to replenish. I've tried using the battery analogy with friends and family but find that banking works better (says a lot about me and my family!) so here goes with me trying to explain how the cost-benefit ratio and pacing all fit into the energy bank.

Imagine that prior to getting Covid, you had £100 in a bank. Covid took some people's bank balances down to £99 and others to £1. Gradual recovery from Covid saw the bank balances return, at varying speeds, to £100. For LCers, despite recovering from the Covid-19 infection, the bank balance has never gone back to £100 and may never do so. The optimum bank balance that LCers can reach with current knowledge, techniques and so on is £60. Instantly, you can see that even on the very best day, an LCer is 40% behind what they used to be and non LCers who can achieve £100 relatively easily. On the very worst days, LCers can have only £1 in the bank, making us 99% less than what we once were.

"Just try and build the balance up," is a common comment. The answer is, "That's what we are trying to do with pacing, cost-benefit ratios and so on." No matter what we do, the balance is not going over £60 for any LCer who has not recovered from LC and many of us see the £60 target as a mountain still to climb. The spending is physical, emotional, mental and spiritual and, where most people without LC can have a couple of days of rest or a good night's sleep to have their bank balance shooting back to £100 even from £1, that just doesn't/can't happen with LC.

A day spent in A and E with my father recently left my bank balance at £1. I was emotionally and mentally drained at the end of it, so much so that I forgot how to walk up the stairs, mid-step. I was staring at my feet and having no clue how to carry on upwards. I knew where I was going and what I was going to do when I got there but I couldn't figure out how to carry on up those stairs until my husband coached me through it. I would put my energy bank at £1, based on that and the hoarseness, the stammering and the incomprehension that went with it. I had a good night's sleep afterwards but my energy levels didn't zip back up. That's not how LC works. The hours of stress and strain in that one day meant it took me four days to be able to not have to sleep for up to five hours in the afternoon, to be able to participate in conversations and for my joint pain to die down. Even then, I wasn't back at my £60 optimum, it was closer to £40. A couple of weeks with grandchildren, punctuated by two long drives and two long coach trips had me in bed for a week afterwards, in a lot of physical pain with the fatigue rendering me useless. Again, though, despite the bedrest, my energy bank was only registering a £35 balance at the end of that week.

I think what I'm trying to explain is that all the pacing and technique planning in the world can't stop a LC crash coming and there's no such thing as a quick rebound from the symptoms. A lot of tears flow every time, when I'm not too fatigued to cry, because I observe the impact my low or negative bank balance has on those around me. I can't move effortlessly from one family crisis to another any more. I always have to choose who to help and who to let down and end up letting even more people down when the LC kicks in afterwards. There's the non LCer expectation that a good sleep or a rest will suddenly put the bank balance back up to where it should be and the exasperation with me when it doesn't work that way. The bank balance has to be drip fed, £1 by £1, and any withdrawals while re-building the balance last longer than they would without LC. I hope that explains the whole energy bank and deficit thing that happens with LC. *The Long Covid Self Help Guide* explains the energy bank very well in terms of a battery - it may be worth a look!

Exercise. It is widely accepted that exercise can improve physical health and mental wellbeing with the release of the hormone Serotonin into the brain. The right exercises can help improve lung capacity and general overall fitness levels. The benefits are enormous and should make regular exercising a no-brainer, a slam dunk in things to do to help with LC. So why is it so hard to do?

Motivation is a big one, personally. I am a lazy individual anyway, always have been, and the thought of exercising when all my joints are flaring and I am exhausted doesn't add to the thrill of wanting to exercise. I've read the motivational tracts on finding the exercise that you enjoy and come up empty. How I manage is by setting a step target each day and trying to achieve it. It's currently a pathetic 2,500 steps but on a bad LC day, even that is impossible, with me lucky to make 100 steps.

My local LC rehab team has devised an exercise programme that runs for an hour, twice a week for six weeks. One of the physios running it is superb, always listens and cares about the individuals in his classes, rather than worrying about ticking the boxes of how many attend and how quickly they can be crossed off the exercise part of the rehab programme. This was an excellent motivator for me and I attended all the classes, either in person or over Zoom. The drawback is that the programme that was designed from on high is a one size fits all session, meaning there are parts that not everyone can do and not everyone's individual needs can be catered for, making the classes not perhaps as useful as they may have been. The attitude of some of the instructors stank, frankly. They'd shrug if I couldn't do a particular thing and concentrate on those who could, which wasn't a huge amount of help to those of us who may have needed something gentler or more attuned to what our LC was letting us do. But a huge BRAVO to the ones who did care and did try to cater for everyone within the constraints set for them. I'm glad I did the classes and, for a while, I felt fitter for it.

The problem with adding exercise to the day when you have LC is that it feeds the fatigue and Post Exertional Malaise elements, sometimes stoking those fires so high that for days afterwards, nothing more than getting in and out of bed is possible. I always feel it kind of negates the point of trying to get fitter if it leaves me more exhausted and broken than I was before the activity! I can't say that one kind of exercise is better or worse for LC in my experience. I think it's a very individual thing, just like LC. I've found what's working for me at the moment and fully accept that it probably isn't the best in terms of results but I feel fitter than I did pre-Covid, even if my fatigue levels are so much higher. Given all the benefits touted for exercise, I try to keep plugging away with the steps but not beating myself up if I don't make it on certain days.

The advice I can offer is to find what suits you as a LCer and what works for you within your LC symptoms. Don't get pushed beyond your LC limits by others, no matter how well-meaning, and take each step as a victory. One thing I know without a doubt is that movement is key in everything LC. Stopping moving pushes you into a longer malaise, further fatigue, more brain fog so even a minimal number of steps in a room every day, a few arm swings here and there, a couple of neck exercises keeps movement present. When I had Covid for the third time, I forced myself to walk down the road most days and, as the Covid wore off, I could get a little bit further round the block. I can't guarantee it went sooner or was less severe because I was attempting movement and exercise every day but I know I felt better quicker and that was something I had done very differently to the first two infections. Any exercise, any movement helps, in my opinion.

In *The Long Covid Handbook,* Gez Medinger suggests the way forward with exercise is to avoid being completely sedentary but stay within personal limits. He also identifies that a generally accepted rule for LC is ensuring the heart rate remains below 60% of its maximum. I feel this information needs to be shared with exercise organisers, be they physiotherapists, specialist leaders or general keep kit instructors, because most classes take individuals way over that 60% and for LCers, this could be dangerous. As ever, self-awareness and spreading awareness is the way forward.

<u>F is for...</u>

Fatigue. I don't mean the 'I didn't sleep well' tiredness. I don't mean the 'What a tiring day, I've been so busy,' tiredness. Fatigue is to tiredness what the Great Wall of China is to Tower Bridge, in that you can acknowledge, admire and notice the latter, but the former defies description in its vastness, overtaking and consuming everything around it. A very common perception of fatigue is that it's just tiredness or laziness and everyone gets tired. Fatigue is not tiredness. Fatigue is when you physically cannot put one foot in front of another. Fatigue is when your brain shuts down so you can't think or speak coherently. Fatigue is when you can't understand what is being said to you because your brain just won't hear and process the words. Fatigue is when you want to cry with exhaustion but you just can't muster the energy to do so. Fatigue is like being encased in old, heavy armour. Fatigue is like walking through quicksand covered in treacle - you get nowhere with it. There's no way around it, no way through it, no escaping it.

Long Covid means I have to factor in fatigue to every plan, every day, all the time. That's not to say I am fatigued every day any more. I was in the beginning and it was hell for me and those around me. Getting in the shower was the only achievement I had in a day and getting out again was a saga in itself. I have recovered enough and have learnt enough about my body's signals that I can 70% accurately predict a fatigue crash. This helps in some ways because I can plan accordingly. Sometimes. Sometimes, the outside influences in life means I can predict a crash but can't do anything about it other than fall headlong into it because of the commitments I have. "Change the commitments then," I am told. "Stop doing so much. Think of yourself." Sometimes, that can be done but sometimes, it just can't. "Sorry, dad, I can't come to the hospital to sit with you through chemotherapy because I know I'll get fatigued afterwards," is not a sentence I am ever prepared to say. Nor is, "Sorry, love, I know you're depressed and suicidal but I can't take the time to listen because I will be fatigued afterwards." Nor is, "Sorry, I can't watch your sports day because I'll get fatigued." You get the picture without another thousand examples.

And so the fatigue bus rolls on. In a way, the planning means an adaptation, a resignation, an acceptance because LC life cannot be lived without it. The fatigue isn't going anywhere so I can choose to plan around it, as much as I can in my circumstances, or I can give in to it and exist with LC, not moving further than the bedroom and the bathroom. And, believe me, there's days like that still, where the stairs are insurmountable and the bathroom is 300 miles away and I can't think or speak properly. Understanding eludes me, ironically as does sleep. Fatigue doesn't mean you can just sleep it off. Very often, sleep just won't come or if it does, it's in small, nonrestorative patches.

What's the answer? Honestly, they don't have it yet. The Chronic Fatigue service can offer a lot of helpful suggestions and tips but where LC is so varied, only the individual can work through and find something - anything! - that helps them. LC has such a varied effect on its victims that there is no clear, definitive answer to any of the symptoms, fatigue included. I'm still searching, still looking for that definitive answer that may never come but trying out different things to manage my fatigue so that I can function, if not on a daily basis, on a higher percentage than not functioning at all.

Frustration. Hand in hand like the twins from *The Shining* come frustration and guilt. Interchangeably, one leads to the other. Arguably, that's true for everyone, with or without LC, and I couldn't honestly say it never happened to me prior to LC. It did, big time. However, LC seems to have magnified the power of the evil twins because I feel more frustrated and more guilty every extra day that I have LC. I can't function the way I did pre-LC and it frustrates me. Every time I have to say no to an activity or spending time with someone because I am just too fatigued to even think, it's frustrating. Having to plan every microsecond around LC is frustrating, especially when it still all goes wrong despite the minutiae being planned microscopically. Even writing this book has taken way longer than I ever planned because I just don't have the ability to concentrate for long periods of time or don't have even small chunks of brain capacity for days on end. Taking the words and thoughts out of my head and putting them onto paper has taken a ridiculous amount of time to achieve.

It's not just me who gets frustrated. Family are tired of hearing, "because of my Long Covid" at the start or end of a reason why I can't do something and even quote it back at me as, "I suppose because of the Long Covid, you can't..." And I feel guilty that days out are curtailed, that activities are cut short or just don't happen or that long-awaited trips are abandoned due to the uninsurable health issues caused by LC, along with the need to make a two week trip into a month long trip to accommodate my pacing needs and patterns, rendering such trips unaffordable and impossible. It is so frustrating that I am either holding my family back due to LC or that I can't participate in their activities and have to watch from the sidelines, making me so unhappy for them and myself. There's no way of expressing how upsetting it is to have plans with others, only for them to be scuppered by joint pain flares and/or fatigue that mean all I can do is crawl around my bedroom in a lot of pain for an inestimable amount of time.

As there is no sign of my LC abating, although I can't argue it hasn't improved using all the techniques in the LC toolbox, the frustration grows daily. With frustration comes guilt and anger at myself. It's all very destructive emotionally and very wearing for everyone else too, as well as frustrating. The lack of knowledge about potential recovery times, as well as the lack of knowledge about LC itself is at the heart of it all. There's no magic fix - or any fix at all. It's all the dreaded 'wait and see' approach that hospital consultants seem so fond of. It's too new to have any concrete answers so the ongoing state of limbo just adds to the daily, growing frustration at the insurmountability of this illness.

Another aspect of the frustration is the believability of LC. There are so many people out there who believe genuine LCers are just swinging the lead to either get out of things they don't want to do or to try and get benefits from the government. And, most annoying and frustrating of all, there are the people who don't have LC but who have seen it as a great way to get 6 months paid sick leave from work, miraculously being recovered enough to go back on the day their pay is due to drop to half pay. Any genuine LCer can tell you that is impossible. LC doesn't work that way and such precise planning just can't happen. Well, the planning can but the reality is a whole different animal. It's those LC fakers that make it difficult for genuine LCers to be taken seriously, as well as taking up valuable places in LC recovery programmes that could go to a genuine sufferer. It makes me want to scream with frustration. I have certainly ranted long and hard about it but, much as I would like to, I have no control over the actions of others who act so detrimentally towards those of us who genuinely need the help.

Frustration has many facets. Others get frustrated with me and my LC. I get frustrated with others' lack of understanding and the lack of knowledge, longevity and curability of LC. Coupled with guilt, frustration is a huge part of LC that is proving almost impossible to overcome.

<u>G is for...</u>

Grief. Grief is a non-physical symptom of LC for me. I spend a lot of time close to tears grieving for what I have lost and that makes it hard to look forward and pull positives from what I have at this moment in time. Trying to compose a letter for my daughter would have taken ten minutes tops pre LC. Now, it takes the best part of two hours, with the need to re-read, edit, scream mentally for words that just won't come and remain unsatisfied that the job wasn't done as could as it could have been and feel that my having LC has let her down. And that brings on the grief for what is lost. I can't seem to get beyond the grieving for what I was, what I might have been and for everything that I now cannot do thanks to LC.

Grief feels heavy. It's a burden that weighs me down daily, every time I can't leap from one thing to another, be that mentally, physically or emotionally. It grieves me when I have to rest after a drive that has been mentally taxing, making overnight trips a terror filled nightmare of having an LC crash (not a car crash!) in the middle of a motorway because I have pushed the limits of my new capabilities way too far. The planning of anything brings grief because I initially plan for the way things were, so the timings, the activities, even the sleeping arrangements are in place. Then I think about what is realistic to achieve with LC and they all have to change. A trip that could be a swift day trip now has to involve a two night hotel stay, while the expeditions on the trip now have to be broken down into 3 days of a bit of activity with a lot of resting in the hotel room for me and boredom for my companion. Anyone travelling with me has to fit around my capabilities or lack thereof. And that grieves and frustrates me. So much has had to change for everyone because of my LC and it breaks my heart to think of it. LC has brought genuine loss to my life and I weep in grief and despair. It's impossible to stay positive all the time and some days, you just don't want to keep picking yourself back up so give in and wallow in the grief. It happens. Cue the guilt.

Guilt. Guilt is another huge factor in my LC life. I feel guilty every day because I can't do what I could before Covid-19 hit. That means I can't help and support everyone in my life the way I used to for extended periods of time. The kinder they are about my lack of ability, the more guilty I feel because it is like I am letting them down. I feel guilty that I can't be a 'proper' grandmother to my grandbabies. The numbness and sudden arm weakness mean I am terrified to pick them up in case I drop them. This is fine if it's a hug, because I can do that seated or on my lap. But if they cry, I am scared to lift them up in case they fall. The fatigue means I don't have the stamina to play their games for long and, whilst they are happy to cuddle for a while on the sofa with the TV, it feels intrinsically wrong to be doing that with them.

The brain fog plays a big part in the guilt too. Come evening, it is guaranteed that if someone wants to talk to me, I find my attention drifting away, sometimes with a complete incomprehension of what they are saying and so I spend a lot of time hoping I'm saying the right thing in response or that my facial expressions are appropriate. It happens throughout the day too but the evenings are the worst. And I feel terrible about it because they deserve better from me but I just don't have it to give any more.

Fatigue impacts my life hugely in the guilt stakes too. I just can't keep pace with my family any more on days out or on holiday. Day 3 is always a point of fatigue, joint pain flares and bad brain fog, even with the best pacing and planning, so it is a day written off to LC. If my husband wants to visit 3 sightseeing attractions in a day, I'm now only capable of going to one if it's a good day. I feel so bad about them having to adjust to my pace or work their plans around me. An alternative of extending a holiday or sending people off alone is unappealing but often the latter is the only practical way. Extended, longer holidays equal higher costs and, in the current economic climate, that is a huge no-no. LC is already costing us money because I can't work, so the thought of spending more to literally accommodate LC is intolerable. Days out and holidays are a compromised, half the time experience now - if I even manage to go on them - and the guilt-trip every time is a crushing burden to bear.

"Don't feel guilty," is a phrase I hear a lot but I do. It's *my* illness, *my* fatigue and *my* brain fog that has been forced upon those I care about and it disrupts our interactions and our plans. No one had any choice about it and I feel so guilty about the effect it is having on our daily life. Talking therapy helps but the guilt remains.

<u>H is for...</u>

Hair loss. About two months after being diagnosed with LC, I noticed that more and more hair was coming out of my head each time I brushed it. Not enough to be leaving clumps on pillows or anything like that but enough to notice a huge mat in the hairbrush after each use. My hair thinned considerably but, as I am lucky enough to have quite a thick crop, it wasn't instantly noticeable to anyone other than me. I couldn't work out what was going on. I mean, what did hair have to do with LC? It was only talking to the physio at my Covid rehab assessment appointment that I became aware that it is yet another LC symptom.

Luckily, the rate of loss seems to have calmed down a lot and, whilst my hair is thinner than it used to be, at least I'm not shedding swathes like I was two years ago.Occasionally, I go through a brief period where large amounts come out again but then it suddenly stops. There seems to be no trigger for it to happen. It just happens. Now I know it's part of LC and also that it stops after about a week these days, I am less concerned about it.

Hallucinations. I'll stand up and admit that I have hallucinations as a result of LC. I've had the CT scan on my brain, as well as an MRI, and there's nothing untoward going on up there that they can see. My hallucinations don't appear every day, week or month but they do have a pattern of sorts. When I hit the post-exertional malaise and fatigue stage of LC before the supercrash, I start to get strange things appearing in my line of sight. Or just outside my line of sight but enough to be aware and be thinking, "What's that?" Very much like the *Listen* episode of Dr Who, where he ruminates on things in the corner of your eye, that's how the hallucinations are for me. After the initial "What's that?" moment, I know they aren't real and am aware that I am hallucinating and that I need to get to lie down pretty swiftly because a supercrash is only a few minutes away.

They don't always happen before a crash so it's not a guaranteed way of detecting an oncoming crash. But a crash always appears after my hallucinations, so I sometimes get a warning of the impending disaster that I have learned to heed. They are mostly harmless flickers on the periphery of my vision but it can be dangerous if I am driving because my human instinct is to swerve away from something I may hit. The knock on effect of this is to make me nervous about driving, especially if it is a longer trip or a shorter trip requiring a lot of concentration, such as to a new place I've not visited before. Does this mean I should give up driving? My initial feeling is no, because there is no regularity or frequency to the hallucinations and they are quite rare. The medical profession isn't terribly helpful either on that question. When asked, they suggest that it is up to me, as there is nothing obviously wrong with the way my brain is firing. A heavy dose of disbelief is always evident in the very few discussions I have had on the topic of hallucinations and driving.

Day to day, I don't find they affect me at all, apart from being a handy warning of LC crashes to come. They don't scare me, just more take me by surprise occasionally. I think I have had two instances of hallucination in the last seven months, so there's no kind of urgency about them. Plus I can tell that they are hallucinations. The corner of the eye ones are the trickiest but a blue gremlin jumping out in front of me? Yeah, I've got that one logged as not really there! I wonder if it's my brain trying to rewire and this is one of the side effects of it. Or maybe my body setting up a warning system so I can be ready to lie down when the crash arrives? Either way, hallucinations are not something I fear. I can't argue that I welcome them but they just are what they are - another LC symptom for me.

Heart issues. I was due to fly to Seville for a few days' holiday - the first time ever that my husband of 31 years and I would have been abroad together, just the two of us. 10 hours before the flight, I had a crashing pain in my chest and back, like I was being squeezed in a vice. Cue breathing problems, pain in my neck and shoulder and a very swift ambulance ride to the hospital for a battery of heart related tests. Six hours later, I was released with the good news that they didn't think it had been a heart attack but they couldn't entirely rule it out so I could not be certified fit to fly. I put it down to stress, anxiety, you name it but not once did it occur to me (or them!) that it was in any way LC related.

A few days after the Seville non-event, on 26 February 2023, The Mail on Sunday published an article by Ethan Ennals about LC and the research that seems to indicate that it doubles the chances of major heart troubles starting. The theme of the research seems to be that the doctors involved in the study were finding that LC was causing inflammation and hidden clots in blood vessels, leading to heart troubles. Dr Malcolm Finlay, a consultant cardiologist, was quoted as saying, "Covid appears to have some direct impact on the heart," and went on to say, "It's important that we continue to follow these heart problems…to see what the long-term effect of Long Covid is."

I found this both concerning and great. Concerning because I don't want to add heart problems to my ever-growing list of LC problems but great because it means I can ask the GP to take it seriously and get some investigations done. It's a shame I feel I have to legitimise my request for help but at least there is now some very public research to wave at GPs, cardiologists etc to get it ruled out, if nothing else.

I had a cardiac monitor, ECGs, blood tests (yes, more!) and a blood pressure monitor all booked in and ready to go. The results were typical LC results. The cardiac monitor showed nothing abnormal and neither did the ECG, apart from the fact that my heart was racing on occasions with no obvious cause. The blood tests were inconclusive. The blood pressure monitor showed, that throughout the day, I was reaching stroke level blood pressure every time my heart raced. Still not worth seeing a cardiologist, apparently.

Chatting to a friend of mine who does not have LC, she told me Covid affected the electrical signals in her heart, giving her resting heart rates of up to 165 beats per minute! She is due to have cardiac ablation surgery as a result, with the hope of being able to walk fast or dance again. This is proof that heart and Covid are linked so, by extension, the heart and LC can also be linked. Being aware that LC can affect the heart is a big thing to be aware of and to make medical professionals aware of. Most know very little about LC because it is such a wide ranging thing. Because the knowledge about it is scanty but expanding every day, it's almost an onus on the LC sufferer to keep abreast of research developments and try to pass on any information to the medics. Whether they will look further into it is very much an individual thing, I find.

Hoarseness. Medically known as dystonia, hoarseness comes and goes and makes me look like a particularly bad actress when I'm hoarse at the start of a sentence and speaking normally by the end of it. I know when I'm getting tired or a crash is on the way because I suddenly go from a normal voice to sounding like a chain smoking troll living under the bridge. And it stays that way until the fatigue or crash clears, which is great fun for all those around me but not so good if I'm on a serious phone call and suddenly change voice or am with a particularly deaf relative. Seriously, though, dystonia is another very handy warning tool for me that an LC crash is coming and I need to try to stop and rest. Obviously, that's not always possible but it goes back once again to listening to what my body is telling me and trying to obey the cues it is giving me. If I get the chance to rest, I bounce back a lot quicker than if I can't or don't rest. Whilst the croaking can be inconvenient, it is also incredibly helpful.

Hyperacceleration. Another of LC's many talents seems to be the ability to hyperaccelerate medical outcomes that were years away. When I experienced pain in every - literally every - joint in my body at exactly the same time, I saw a consultant rheumatologist. A lovely man, who was calm and accepting of LC as a thing, he did a battery of blood tests, X rays and so on. Apparently, Heberden's nodes had appeared on every one of my fingers at the same time, apparently a very unusual phenomenon. Osteophytes had appeared on some of my vertebrae, seemingly overnight.

As usual, the tests were negative and I'm still grateful that no nasty shocks emerged. However, that led to the obvious question of why? There seemed to be no explanation other than LC's influence over my body. The rheumatologist's theory was hyperacceleration. My response was, "Huh?" His thought was that I was due all these delights anyway in life but not for another 20-30 odd years and LC had somehow accelerated my inevitable decline. Looking at my fingers and the scans of my vertebrae, I can see how the hypothesis could be valid. It makes me wonder if any organs such as heart, lungs or liver have been artificially decimated prematurely and exactly what LC is capable of. For now, though, it's another sigh and another bad mark for LC.

Hypersensitivity. One LC thing I have noticed that affects me internally and externally is how hypersensitive my body has become. I'm not talking mentally or emotionally - that is a whole different topic! Physically, I am feeling pain quicker and sharper than before and it seems more extreme. The smallest knock into something and I have a bigger 'ow' reaction than before but also a bigger bruise. Blood tests have shown that there is nothing wrong with clotting etc so it is down to hypersensitivity. Interestingly, my senses haven't suddenly become super spidey senses - quite the opposite, they've all dulled with LC. It is the body that is now on hyper reaction alert.

My GP confirmed the hypersensitivity theory when I went to him with a severe allergic reaction to the third lot of blood pressure pills, having had a less severe but nonetheless allergic reaction to two other sets. I asked him why I now seem to get side effects to any new medicine (by new I mean post LC new prescriptions). He told me that the body is now hypersensitive to many things and it is currently an emerging symptom of LC. That made me feel better in a way because, in the case of prescription medicine, it's not a case of me reading the side effects sheet and developing them in a hypochondriac way. The fact that my eyeballs had swollen should have proven that to me but it's nice to feel it's not down to a desire for attention.

Loud noises make me jump more and my heart beats faster when I hear them. This is despite me not hearing as well as before LC - go figure. I have a couple of food allergies and, again, my reaction to them if ingested by accident (garlic is in almost everything I don't make myself!) is stronger than pre LC. My fingers are numb a lot of the time but as soon as something sharp goes near them, it's intense pain. I have a lot more examples but you get the picture.

LC has put my body on high alert and it's trying to reject anything internally it can't cope with by reacting in a painful and consistent way. A suggestion has been to try to engage the parasympathetic nervous system to try and calm it down. A lot easier said than done and no fellow LCer has found that is a permanent solution or, in the majority of people I have spoken to, any kind of solution at all. No physiological change has been shown in the people who have been through tests for it but it's there, it exists now. A heavy dose of steroids has solved my latest hypersensitive reaction to medication but it would be good to think that one day, I may not need steroids to calm my body down. I'm hoping a solution comes quickly or my body adapts because at the moment, every day is like being a hyper wired meerkat on the alert for a new predator. And I don't like being a meerkat!

I is for...

Immune system. It seems as if there are two schools of thought on whether Covid affects the immune system. One school goes down the definitely not route, as there's no concrete evidence that the immune system is compromised by the initial infection. The other school has a modicum of research available that seems to indicate that Covid has affected the immune system but that this only shows up in individuals with LC. Personally, I subscribe to the second school of thought because I have never caught so many bugs or infections as I have since getting LC. Others in my LC group say they have never been as sickly as they are now.

After any trip out, mask or no mask, I am guaranteed to have a cough or cold within the week. The hint of a stomach bug in the family has me dashing for the bathroom in the most unbecoming way. The more serious illnesses are concerning. The recent Influenza A outbreak had me hospitalised over the Christmas period, having fallen victim to the infection. What is the answer? I'm boosting myself with multivitamins, keeping hydrated, trying to exercise more and trying to follow any and all guidelines for boosting the immune system. I can't say I've been hugely successful, as the illnesses keep plaguing me and when they strike, what was a simple 24 hour thing now knocks me out for a week, thanks to the long reach of LC.

There's not enough research to conclusively prove that the immune system is broken by Covid and even less to say whether it is recoverable. All I know is that I am a believer in LC decimating the immune system as well. A member of an LC group I belong to now makes no antibodies in response to injections for things like flu, tetanus etc. He has been tested and retested and, sure enough, 4 weeks after a vaccination, the body has produced no antibodies and his immune system is wrecked. He was fine prior to Covid so whilst it cannot be down to LC, it could certainly be claimed that it was as a result of the Covid infection, giving rise to the theory that people with LC can have compromised immune systems.

Inflammation. In the Mail on Sunday's article about LC causing heart issues, there was a nod to inflammation, buried within the main cardiac feature. Research carried out by the Global Remote Research Scholars Program demonstrated that diagnostics tests prove LC sufferers have consistently high levels of inflammation body-wide, despite it being potentially years since the initial Covid infection. The swollen hands and joints, the head pressure from swollen sinuses, the jaw ache from the swelling in the neck and glands, the costochondritis that feels like a heart attack, the knees that crack with each movement are all caused by inflammation, the wicked uncle of LC.

I have had inflammation in at least one part of my body every day since I caught Covid-19 in August 2021. Taking anti-inflammatories like ibuprofen or naproxen long term can give you ulcers or stomach bleeds so it can be a bit of a no win situation. Daily, I choose between the pain or the potential ulcers. Thanks to LC, there is no end date in sight for this decision making. One natural solution I have found that helps me is a gummy containing ginger and turmeric. I'd be lying if I said it cures all the inflamed parts of my body. It doesn't but it does take the edge off on days when the inflammation pain is already tolerable and means I can avoid the NSAIDs for that time. Long term answer? I don't think there is one yet, any more than there is a solution for the inflammation caused by such things as osteoarthritis. It's more a case of managing it than curing it.

It's a thing, is it? A consultant gynaecologist asked me that. Ladies, you will know what I mean when I say he was one of those gynaes who seem to despise women (or maybe it was just me!) so make you wonder why they became a gynaecologist. As you can probably guess, things weren't going well at the appointment anyway. He was throwing information at me, not listening to my responses and I was finding it more and more difficult to form thoughts and articulate them, due to the LC brain fog. As he huffed impatiently, I told him the reason I was having trouble explaining myself was because I had Long Covid. The sneer down the nose look, followed by the words, "Long Covid? It's a thing, is it?" simultaneously made my blood boil and made me burst into tears. He wasn't expecting the tears and sighed, moving straight on to something else, brushing over the whole LC question. Here's what I wish I could have said at the time.

Yes, LC is real. Yes, it's intangible. Yes, I know there are people out there swinging the lead but I'm not one of those people. I wish I was because then fatigue and compensating for it wouldn't be ruling my life. I wish I was making it up because then I wouldn't be fighting it day in, day out with no let up. I wish I was making it up because I wouldn't be dealing with the tuts and the eye rolls from people when I mention it as a reason for why I can't do a particular thing at a particular moment. I wish I was making it up because then my brain would function like it used to and I wouldn't be screaming mentally with frustration. I wish I was making it up because then I wouldn't feel so bloody awful all the time. But I'm not making it up. It's like all the backaches and headaches that you can't see but are real.

Idleitis is another thing I have been accused of. Constantly having to lie down to rest after the smallest exertion. Gazing blankly around without any understanding of what is going on around me. Saying I can't work because I can't concentrate long enough or am too tired to do so for even a few hours. Bone idle are the words often thrown my way, along with sponger. For the record, I am not on benefits and, knowing the ridiculous hoops my disabled daughter has to jump through to get any kind of help from the 'system', I know there is minimal hope for many LC sufferers because so much about LC is intangible. Honestly, I'd love to be idle because that would mean I was capable of doing the things in the first place. But, for now, I'm not and I have a new year's resolution not to let these critics get to me. I know my own truth.

Another consultant, when asking what I did for a job and hearing I hadn't worked since LC struck, glanced at me, sighed and said, "That long? Oh my, my." Which looks okay in print because print can't show the critical tone in which it was said, along with the immediate dismissal thereafter of anything I had to say about my (for once!) LC unrelated issue. Not a direct "It's a thing, is it?" comment but as good/bad as one.

I despair of any long term support for the majority of LCers because of these pervading attitudes. Due to the nature of LC and the broad spectrum of medical specialities that it seems to invade, there's too wide a range for all the specialists to be an expert in their field and in LC and how it applies to their field. Because of the gamut of symptoms, it would be nigh on impossible to have a consultant in LC. Add to that the potentially temporary (ha!ha!) nature of LC, there would be no point in training doctors up for it. It would, however, be good for everyone to have an LC awareness training of some sort so that, even though there are undoubted fakers out there, comments like these from medical 'professionals' to their patients could be avoided.

So yes, **IT IS A THING** and to have hospital consultants suggest otherwise is personally disheartening and professionally damaging to all those who, like me, are just trying to deal with it, overcome it and are fighting to be believed. Fighting to be taken seriously. Fighting to get help. Fighting for research into a cure. Fighting just to get well again.

I.Q. Before Covid, my IQ was 148 and I felt that I was quite bright. IQ shouldn't be used as a measure for everyday life because common sense matters more and is far more relevant but I wondered, for interest, if the brain fog of LC was affecting my IQ at all. I did a few online tests (not the official Mensa ones, I hasten to add) and my IQ is now 102! Quite a drop, I felt and I was quite shocked to have dropped 46 points. I juggled theories in my mind - it wasn't an official Mensa one; was it brain fog meaning I didn't understand things that I could understand quite easily before; was it simply down to the fact that I couldn't concentrate for the full 30 minute test and so was just clicking answers at random by the end? I didn't have the answer so decided to try a different test the following day to see if the results would be similar. On the Mensa workout, I scored 9 out of 18 (ouch!). On another IQ testing site on a different day when I was feeling fresh and quite 'with it', I scored 86%, where the average score is 51.1%, with my incorrect answers being the total guesses where my brain wouldn't do the maths for me. Yet another attempt on a day where I had been concentrating a lot before taking the test and was feeling foggy, my IQ was 96.

What conclusions can I reach? I think I have good days and bad and my language skills are definitely better than my maths! As to whether LC and brain fog has affected my IQ, the only conclusion I can draw is that my ability to concentrate affects my IQ scores, not necessarily my general IQ, although I haven't done enough different tests at different times of day and in different stages of brain fog to verify that as a valid conclusion. It will be interesting to keep testing myself to see what happens over the coming months and years on good brain fog days and bad ones. On with that brain training app!

<u>J is for...</u>

Jigsaws. I've never been fond of jigsaw puzzles. They've always appeared too hard (even the 100 piece ones!) and I've had no interest in doing them. Then one of the physios suggested to me to try them as a form of therapy for the brain fog and numbness in my hands, to improve the way my brain is firing and my hand/eye coordination. Starting with the basic children's 16 pieces, I found it almost impossible to complete a jigsaw at that level. A bit of perseverance and a few bad words took me up to being able to do 49 piece ones, moving up relatively swiftly to 100 pieces in a day. This may sound ridiculous but when the brain isn't sending any signals to help you comprehend the pictures and colours in front of you, believe me when I say it was a major achievement.

I tried and failed to move up to 200, 300 and even 500 pieces. My brain wasn't having it - no thanks, no way. I shelved the puzzles and moved away from jigsaws. I worked with brain training apps on my phone and the Nintendo DS was resurrected for various games and puzzles. I enjoyed them but found I could do some of the activities only if they sparked some kind of interest in me, while others remained forever a mystery my brain refused to unlock. I wondered then about returning to jigsaws with a very specific brief. They had to interest me and they had to be made up of smaller complete pictures joined up, such as 1960's bars of chocolate, rather than one set piece like a cottage in a wood. My brain just shut down at a scene but the smaller complete pieces seemed to be achievable with a lot of effort. I progressed to 200 then 300 pieces puzzles using this criteria. Not fast, not easy, but I did them.

After successfully finishing a 500 piecer, my confidence was knocked when I almost had a panic attack opening a 500 piece that seemed to fulfil my criteria. It had lots of small pictures joining into one and the subject was of interest. So what happened? Why the feeling of being overwhelmed and in a state of panic? Once calm, I tried to work it out. I concluded that, despite it fulfilling my self-determined criteria on one level, it missed them on another. The pieces were very small, making my numb fingers drop them over and over. Whilst the pictures were self contained, they contained a lot of writing in very small print, which my brain just wasn't able to process when in 500 pieces, meaning they made no sense to me. Subconsciously, I shut down because the rewiring hasn't reached that stage yet and panic ensued.

Having solved the problem and to try and rebuild my confidence, I dropped back to a 300 piece very orange dinosaur puzzle. Whilst there was a lot of cursing over the orangeness, the size of the pieces and the lack of a surfeit of tiny information meant my brain could cope again and I relaxed and eventually finished it, confidence restored and a valuable lesson learned on how my brain is still relearning, still rewiring and some things just aren't meant to be, no matter how suitable they first appear. I am now starting a 1,000 piece effort, which has writing on the side of chocolate bars but no swathes of text. It may take months and my four year old granddaughter can still easily outstrip me on the puzzle building front but I feel confidence and a strange kind of peace that I will succeed. Jigsaws can, in my opinion, provide some valuable LC therapy!

Joints. During and after my second dose of Covid-19, I was literally painfully aware that every joint in my body felt as if it was on fire. When I say every joint, I mean every joint. Three joints per finger, per hand, wrists, elbows, jaw, neck, shoulders, hips, knees, ankles, toes - you get the picture. Every movement was agony and being touched by something as delicate as a feather caused more pain. My hands started dropping things and ornaments and eggs were regularly smashed. I was referred to neurology - more of that under N!

Ibuprofen and typical anti-inflammatories, be they pills or gels, just didn't touch it and failed miserably. Nothing controlled the fire. Once the Covid had gone, the joint pain remained so I started researching natural anti-inflammatories and found that ginger, boswellia and turmeric had been recommended across the centuries. Boswellia and I did not get on and some interesting bathroom trips occurred as a result of me taking it. However, a supplement that combined ginger and turmeric turned the pain level down from a 10 out of 10 to about a 5 out of 10. Not a cure but certainly a huge improvement. The medics say there's no end in sight for the joint flares. I still have horrible joint flare up days where it's back to 10 out of 10 but on some days, the pain is down to about a 4 out of 10 with help from my good friends Ginger and Turmeric. I live for those days!

Journaling. It seems bang on the current trend to mention journaling and LC. I see journaling mentioned everywhere as a support to various exercises for mental health and LC is no exception. A quick search on Amazon reveals a variety of LC journals available to document thoughts, feelings and progress within the LC journey. Personally, I can't do journaling. I get too impatient and end up getting very irritated with the whole process of examining my feelings, writing down exactly what I can do right now, where I would like to get to in my journey and so on and so on. I was once told that I have an impatient soul and, in the case of journaling, I can see how this is true! It's just not a thing for me, be it for LC documenting or for other purposes. However, I have spoken to other LCers who have found it really beneficial and have found that documenting the small triumphs of progress along the LC track has given them a huge boost mentally. And good on them - I am always delighted when someone finds something that works for them. My advice, then? Give it a go and see how you get on. Don't beat yourself up if you hate it but see if you love it and, if it works for you, great!

Justification. LC is so intangible that it feels like I constantly have to justify why I am so tired, why I have to stop doing something or just can't do something. The refrain of, "Because I have Long Covid…" trips regularly off my tongue, causing much sighing and eye rolling from family. It's not that I particularly want to keep reminding everyone that I have LC, it's because I feel the constant need to justify the huge changes in me and my abilities. Maybe I shouldn't have to but when you feel like you are constantly letting people down because of your new inability to complete previously achievable tasks or your new found woolly incomprehension of what is being said to you, it's almost a compulsive need to shout, "I'm sorry! I don't want me to be like this either!" Having eyes rolled and comments like, "I expect you're off to lie down again, aren't you?" thrown your way pushes the urge to justify your actions way past where it reasonably should be. And that's probably on me rather than those making the comments because I haven't accepted it fully myself. Reasonably then, how can I expect my family to accept the 'new' me without lashings of self-justification from yours truly?

I have this need to justify why I am being so useless compared to pre-Covid days because I haven't fully accepted what has happened to me. If I can't accept it, I cannot expect those around me to accept it, although I feel everyone's life would be more peaceful if they did. In the case of meeting new people, the LC conversation inevitably happens because I crave their understanding. It would be a step too far to say I crave their sympathy but I really do desire their understanding in order to avoid many of the situations I encountered in my early LC days. If they believe in LC, then my attempt at self- justification is met with comprehension and more productive exchanges can happen. Yes, doctors and medics, I am talking about you! If they don't believe in LC, well, no justification speech in the world will change their view that I am a clumsy, lazy thickie. Thanks to some good psychological input from the local talking therapy service, I am coming to the conclusion that that attitude is on them, not me. The need to justify who I am now hasn't left me and my little parrot phrase of, "Because of my Long Covid…" is probably here to stay for the foreseeable future. Annoyingly for everyone, including me.

K is for...

Kindness. Kindness matters. Kindness from friends and family, kindness from medical professionals and kindness to yourself. Kindness lifts the spirits. Kindness calms the spirits. Kindness makes everything feel a bit better and LC more bearable. Unfortunately, sometimes kindness is in short supply, bringing me down mentally and emotionally. Unkindness often dominates many encounters and pushes me down the depression ladder, resulting in me mentally writing off the day, week in and week out. It is so destructive because it makes me lose hope in others and in my abilities. What is heartbreaking is that unkindness continues unabated from others. On a more positive note, when someone is kind, it's like the sun comes out and I feel lifted, even though it can bring me to tears because it's so unusual. A hospital consultant once said to me, "People aren't very kind to you, are they?" which gave me a lot of food for thought.

I have come to realise that I have no control over the kindness of others but I can be kind to myself in unlimited situations, in unlimited thoughts and for unlimited time. I can give myself the space and time I need to deal with LC. I can stop the self criticism and the self destructive thoughts. I can give myself a break from the guilt and the frustration. And when I do, I feel better. I feel calmer. I feel happier. I don't always get it right but when I am kind to myself, I smile more and I breathe easier. It's a long term project but one I am glad to be working on.

Knowledge. In 1597, Francis Bacon declared "Knowledge itself is power," in his work *Meditationes Sacrae*. Thomas Edison and Albert Einstein have quoted him and it's quite a common theme in many spy films, books and so on. It's true of LC as well. There is no one overarching expert in LC worldwide, so it is up to me and my fellow LCers to gather our own knowledge, evidence and research to present to the medical professionals in the hope of getting help. It's important not to be afraid to say, "I need to show you this," and present your knowledge to them. Normally unafraid to express my opinions, I have always, inexplicably, become quiet and a nodding dog when faced with medics and bowed to their instant dismissals of me. WIth LC, where I can't string a sentence together a lot of the time, it's a real challenge. What I have found helped with some (not all!) of the medics is the presentation in written form of indefatigable proof of what I am saying to them, be that an article or factsheet downloaded, a list of published medical papers or whatever. Don't assume this means instant acceptance. In many cases, it will still feel like climbing up a very steep hill backwards but every so often, you get a victory. Knowledge is also self-empowering, Mr Bacon.

<u>L is for...</u>

Listening to your body. Along with finding a baseline, a recurring theme from the Zoom rehab team was listening to the body. The body knows without any input from me what it's capable of on any given day and lets me know in subtle and unsubtle ways. The unsubtle ways are the huge fatigue crashes, the brain fog, the total incapacitation, the emotional breakdowns and so on. I hear those loud and clear! Somehow, I don't think those are the ones the team meant. I think the subtle signs from my body are the ones that will help me manage my fatigue, deal better with my emotional crises and overall handle LC in a more positive way

When I get tired, even mid-sentence, I suddenly go hoarse and my chest starts to feel congested. That's my cue to try to stop or slow down whatever it is I am doing. My eyes suddenly lose focus and almost dip in and out of visual acuity. Mid conversation, it's as if the other person is speaking a language unknown to me that I just cannot understand. If I am holding something, my hands let go with no warning and it's like using a jelly filled rubber glove to try and pick things back up. My back starts spasming and my joints begin to hurt. My lower legs and feet become puffy with swelling. My hands start shaking like I am in drug withdrawal. Each time I've had a major crash, all these signs have been there in the hours and minutes beforehand.

By noticing them and acting upon them, I have managed to cut down on the major crashes. I try to go and rest as soon as one or two symptoms appear. I put anything I am carrying down and don't try to pick it up again while my hands feel numb and go and sit quietly or rest on the bed. By listening to the cues from my body, I can avoid being out of action for up to a week by being out of action for a few hours. It's a hellishly inconvenient way to live life for me and for everyone around me but it's preferable to a full blown crash.

It's also sometimes impossible to act upon the cues. When I'm up in the city, my hoarseness and hand shaking can start but what am I supposed to do? Find a bed in the station or hunker down in the back of a bus? Not possible, trust me. The only option is to carry on, knowing that I need the following days at home to cater for the oncoming crash because the enforced ignoring of the cues means it'll come and it will last.

Loss. I spoke to a lady who had broken her spine and could no longer walk. We opened up a long debate about whether it was mentally tougher to have been physically able to do things and then lose that ability or whether it was mentally tougher to have always had a physical disability. We never really reached a conclusion and it's a conversation that recurs between us every now and then. The loss of a lot of physical and mental capacity due to LC made me revisit these conversations.

It does feel like a loss to be the way I am with LC. I feel that I have lost who I was and there's no sign of re-finding the old me yet. There's always hope because we still don't know if LC will self-resolve for all its victims, unlike for people who have been forced into accepting permanent, life-changing physical disabilities. Is it foolish to cling to hope or more sensible to accept the loss as a permanent feature? I don't know the answer to that one. Should I embrace the loss and rebuild a newer, better version of me based on what I no longer have? These are the 3am questions that keep me awake.

I feel the loss more on some days than others and it's hellish frustrating, anger inducing and sorrowful all at the same time. I feel it the most when I am planning days out or events because I find I plan for the old me and that works out as overplanning for the new me and leaves me incapable after the first event. It's all about the adjusting and adapting but I still feel I have lost a huge part of me. I know I will come to terms with it eventually but for now, there's a big gap where I used to be.

Lungs. I've mentioned the impact of breathlessness etc on my lungs but it's worth more of a mention. When I had influenza A, my lungs felt like they were on fire and the doctor commented about the 'patches' being full of fluid. Prior to Covid, I did not have patches, holes, fluid or anything else on my lungs, so I feel confident in my analysis that my current problems are Covid related. During my third bout of Covid, it felt like I was drowning every time I lay down, no matter how many pillows I used to bolster me upwards. I had an X-ray not long after this Covid session was over and they sent me on my way with no abnormalities detected. Over a month later, I had a call stating that my GP wanted to see me urgently. Much mystified, I went along, to be told that the X-rays had been reexamined and they were worried about a large patch of fluid at the top of my left lung. Two things sprang to mind - over a month before they noticed it and why were they looking again, as no follow up had ever been arranged or discussed? A subsequent X-ray showed the lung to be clear of fluid with no patches, holes etc mentioned or identified. The matter was dropped as the mystery fluid had gone, although my questions still remain unanswered.

No access to a respiratory specialist has ever been offered to me and my lungs. I don't want to use up NHS time unnecessarily but the information, along with most LC information, is inconsistent at best and lacking at worst. Do the patches come and go? Do the holes open up just for flu? What was the fluid in the top of my lung and why was it only in the top of the lung? The answer seems to be that it's gone so it's irrelevant as to why it was ever there. This leaves me in a state of trepidation as to what happens next time I catch Covid 19 or flu or some other respiratory illness. Nothing consistent shows up so no treatment or course of action is forthcoming. LC likes to show no results and so maybe it's all LC just messing about. However, the sensation of drowning and the sensation of not being able to fill the lungs with air or even catch a breath is very real, terrifyingly real.

There are no answers for people who have not been hospitalised with Covid 19 and who have these leftovers from their infection. Is it LC playing or is it real, potentially life-threatening damage? I was told that if I had got on my intended flight with my fluid filled lung, it could have been catastrophic for me, as well as other passengers hoping to reach their destination, as the flight would have had to have diverted due to my lung(s) bursting, collapsing - take your pick - potentially with fatal results. It wouldn't have been good, whatever description you choose. Still not serious enough to see a respiratory specialist because - you guessed it - the fluid isn't there any more.

Getting a straight answer on whether I will be able to fly at some point in the future is impossible. People can fly with lung disease, lung problems and so on as long as it is properly managed. I have nothing on paper stating that this is my case because - yes, again you guessed it - I can't get an appointment with a respiratory specialist because it's 'not necessary' due to the problem being transient or random. Large numbers of LC symptoms are transient and random and don't show up in tests but we LCers know they are real. We know they exist. My seemingly unanswerable question is whether these lung problems of mine are LC related. I have no doubt that they are caused by Covid infections but it's whether the damage is permanent, how I should manage it if it is and whether LC is doing its usual masking and mimicry to throw off results that I need an answer for. Basically, I have no answer to a very big problem.

<u>M is for...</u>

Memory. We've all walked into a room and wondered what we went in there for. Memory is a fragile fairy and LC seems to pull the wings off it and dash it to the floor. Since having LC, my ability to recall a conversation from even five minutes previously has diminished hugely. Huge chunks of conversations, experiences, things I want to ask at appointments just vanish the second after they enter my head. If I am interrupted mid sentence, then it's game over and the point I was making irretrievably lost forever! It could be an age thing but, when I ask fellow LCers, we all seem to be experiencing the same memory problems as part of the brain fog symptom of LC. It can be frightening to be somewhere and suddenly have no clue where you are or why you are there. Even scarier are the scenarios where you forget how to walk up stairs or how to unbolt a door.

I've noticed over my two year LC period that my memory of distant events is improving, so I can recall some childhood memories very vividly. I've been asked how I can remember things from 35 plus years ago so accurately but not what was said to me half an hour ago. I have no answer. Again, you'd hope a neurologist may be interested enough to check the brain for clues but not in my case. Memory is obviously something LC attacks with its brain fog and so maybe my brain is trying to rewire around the blank patches?

I take lists everywhere and I make lists all the time. What was a list of single words has now become an essay around each word because I can't remember why I wrote it down in the first place! My GP is resigned to the notebook being waved his way and a list of items being placed before him, as there have been times when I have gone to visit him and can't recall why. My family are used to seeing lists in strange places with me trailing behind with the words, "Have you seen my list? I can't remember what I'm doing". It's coping strategies that get me through the frustration of not being able to remember things that I know I used to be able to and my lists are a big part of that.

It's scary that my memory doesn't work as well as it did or even very well at all. Along with the rest of LC, there is the huge question of whether or not it ever will again. Is it a permanent thing or will the fog suddenly lift forever? The flip side question is will it continue to deteriorate with every bout of Covid? Will it get to the stage where I recall nothing at all? The LC mimicry has led more than one LCer to be tested for senility because the memory symptoms mimic that of dementia. It's a frightening thing to be experiencing, especially as there seems to be no ongoing improvement, apart from memories of the past which are gaining clarity.

Interestingly, this segment is the one I keep coming back to and adding to. Why? Because I forgot to include things! I'm trying a lot of the memory and mind improvement apps. My favourite is MindPal although I confess to being too mean to pay the subscription which would entitle me to full access and probably an even better experience. I've also resurrected the Nintendo DS from the electronics graveyard and have been buying a variety of brain training games, word training games and so on to play on it, along with puzzle solving ones like Professor Layton. Has any of it made a difference? Honestly, I'm not sure because I have good and bad days with the memory, the words, the general cognition. What I do know is I have a feeling of 'at least I am trying to help myself', which is a good thing to cling to on the darker days.

Mimicry. LC is a far better mimic than any impressionist out there. Symptoms suddenly appear, prompting yet another trip to the GP. I'm sure I now have my own chair in his surgery, poor man! I've had everything from suspected heart attack to excruciating, inexplicable pain to suspected stroke with a whole gamut of things in between. I've been tested, referred and discharged gradually from most of the specialisms because the tests have been negative. It's been LC mimicking the symptoms of each suspected problem, laughing and moving on to something new when the tests come back with a negative result.

When we have chatted, other LCers have reported similar things happening to them. It seems that LC is something it's going to take a long time to pin down and get to the bottom of, in a large part due to the fact that it produces symptoms that belong to other illnesses, diseases etc so is exceptionally good at disguising itself as something else. Which doesn't help us and doesn't help the doctors either because we're all too busy chasing down the wrong rabbit hole while LC decides, "Tonight, Matthew, I'm going to be..."

The more dangerous side of the mimicry is that you don't always take genuine symptoms of other conditions seriously. When my blood pressure went through the ceiling, my very first thought was that LC was just mucking about again with something new and, not wanting to hassle my GP again, I left it for a long time and it was only when the hospital advised to get it regulated urgently because a stroke was imminent that I took it as a real thing, not just the latest LC fakery.

It's certainly a very tricky path to navigate - when is a symptom not a symptom? Is it LC having a laugh or should I get checked out? Every time I catch Covid, LC seems to develop more impressionist skills, making the answer nigh on impossible to get right. I am still looking for that answer and nine times out of ten, I get it wrong. However, I feel that I am trying to aid my recovery and - probably very self delusionally - maybe adding to the LC database of symptoms for the day when more research and knowledge is out there and tests can be more LC targeted.

<u>N is for...</u>

Neurology. Changes to the brain have been officially identified as an effect of Covid so it's important to get seen by a neurologist when you have LC because the changes are literally life changing. One person in my LC group has had MRI scans on his brain before and after contracting Covid. Along with many others, his scans show that the brain has shrunk slightly. This must have some impact on cognition. The LC brain fog feels like parts of the brain have died off and it's trying to rewire itself around the dead bits, often with little success. I need explanations for the inappropriate laughter that bursts out of me when I'm being told or shown terrible things. I want to know why I can no longer juggle four or five things in my head at a time and how I can go back to that ability or whether I will ever have that ability again. How can I get my brain back to where it was or will that never happen? Am I doomed to live with brain fog forever?

I have the misfortune to have a neurologist who is more interested in discharging me so he can tick the 'patient dealt with' box than he is in looking at my brain and what changes have occurred and how to deal with them. He hasn't ordered a CT scan or an MRI on my head and, in fact, has done nothing other than speak on the phone to me. He has certainly never examined me in person and gets impatient when I pause before speaking because I am trying to put words together in my head to reply to his questions. Often, I had to ask him to explain a different way because my brain just wasn't translating the words spoken into comprehension of them. I don't know whether he's a non-believer in LC or whether he's just disinterested in patients. Either way, I have no answers and a building sense of frustration and despair.

A fellow LCer was also referred to a (different) neurologist for her brain fog and LC induced panic attacks when bombarded with information, even if it was just a conversation amongst friends around a table. After two appointments and no scans, she was discharged with a note to the GP that she had made rapid progress, understood her situation and had agreed that nothing further was needed. Sadly, apart from her being discharged, none of it was true. Her GP couldn't do anything because it's the old 'he said, she said' situation and the consultant holds the power, not the patient.

I am going to wait six months and ask for another GP referral and pray I get a different consultant. I can't see any other options open to me. In preparation, I had a private MRI of my brain (open and upright to avoid the claustrophobia. Even then, there was a lot of ugly crying!) I have kept the images so that, fingers crossed, my next attempt at getting help can compare the images from now to images they may take. That's all I can do. I know the consultants are busy and overworked. I know LC is not as life threatening as the majority of other neurological conditions but as brain fog and all its branches are such a major part of LC, you'd think neurologists would be interested, even if only from a research viewpoint. Not all of them, clearly.

Nervous system. It's been proven with LC that the sympathetic part of the autonomic nervous system is stuck in fight or flight mode. This leads to and explains the muscle pain; the fatigue; the brain fog; the insomnia; the palpitations; the racing heart and so on. The parasympathetic part disrupts recovery too so what is the answer? To somehow reset the autonomic nervous system, which is where our good friends the neurologists can come in and help. I'm not lucky enough to have a neurologist who won't stop discharging me because he doesn't believe in LC. However, for those of you who are lucky to have a believer for a consultant, go to them with all these symptoms and ask for help with the reset. It's not a miracle to be worked and may or may not be possible but you have nothing to lose by asking.

For those like me without a sympathetic neurologist, there is still some hope. There's been a lot of research done on the autonomic nervous system and it's a case of trying to find what works (if anything!) for you while hoping to get help from a medical professional. A Google search for 'autonomic nervous system' throws up over 50 million results - way too many to be ploughing through on your own. Even without LC, that's just mind blowing amount of things to deal with. Adding the words 'Long Covid' to the search reduces the numbers to just over 2 million. Still a massive amount but 48 million less! One of the sites I found most useful was https://thedysautonomiaproject.org/lcad/ because it contains links to a variety of other sites that have investigated the effects of LC on the autonomic nervous system and a fact sheet to download to give to your caregiver, as well as a huge amount of information. This one works for me and I still keep dipping in and looking for more and more information.

Calming the nervous system and flipping the sympathetic nervous system switch off is supposed to help. In her book *Breaking Free from Long Covid,* Lucy Gahan includes a chapter on creating a toolkit for dealing with the autonomic nervous system and LC. She offers a variety of techniques such as meditation, diet and cold water therapy. It's well worth a look at the chapter as there are many useful tips, ideas and reasoning, as well as videos to watch on YouTube. There are huge numbers of books, websites etc on stimulating the Vagus nerve, which helps switch off the fight/flight response by activating the parasympathetic nervous system. I've tried and failed to read the books (brain fog!) but it seems to be a growing movement both inside and outside of LC study. A 'watch this space' thing!

What is clear to me is that everyone with LC needs to build a personal toolkit for coping and it's a trial and error thing. Keep plugging away and, if the autonomic nervous system is a key element in LC, then it stands to reason that it could be key in improving LC symptoms too. More research is needed and I'm keeping an eye on sites like the dysautonomia project to hope for advances and ideas that I can implement myself. Anything to improve where I am right now.

New reality. It's hard to adjust and accept a new reality or new me because we just don't know at the present time whether LC is something that will one day just vanish (as per the study where many participants recovered after a year https://www.bmj.com/content/380/bmj-2022-072529) or be curable. At this moment, I am stuck in a new reality because I cannot rely on the old one returning. A new reality where I have to think about every expenditure of energy, where just getting out of bed is sometimes the day's achievement, where anxiety can strike at any second and where a feeling of being crushed and overwhelmed is an almost daily occurrence. It's more than just adapting to something new, it's about adopting a whole new life, a whole new me.

I feel the most important thing to highlight is that it is a reality, not just a hypochondriac's fantasy. It would be so easy to fall into the 'poor little me' way of thinking, where nothing ever gets done or achieved because I'm too busy feeling sorry for myself or thinking I can't do anything. Trying to grasp the positive is not always possible but it's important not to get dragged under by what used to be and who I used to be. The new reality has some good things. I am fitter than I have been in years, despite the fatigue, post exertional malaise etc, because I am making a conscious effort to make my new reality as good as it can be health-wise. I am eating better than I have in years for the same reason. LC has brought my own health into a sharp focus. Rather than completely immersing myself in the problems of others and trying to help solve them as I always have done, I have been forced into looking at my own health and taking some time out for myself to improve what I can concerning my health. I can't do much about LC itself but if I can just get myself as physically, mentally and emotionally fit as I can in this new reality, it gives me a fighting chance of living with LC, potentially for the rest of my life. In fact, I would even venture to say that, whilst I don't like the restrictions and difficulties imposed by LC, it's been a boon to be able to step back and look at my health. My new reality's goal is to be as healthy as I can be and keep plugging away at researching LC and doing my damndest to keep my head above water.

Notepad and pen. An absolute given for me since developing the brain fog part of LC is a notebook and pen. My recall for something from 25+ years ago is still pretty sound but ask me what I saw three minutes ago and I gaze blankly ahead trying to remember. Have I paid that bill? Where am I supposed to be going this afternoon? What was it I wanted to ask the doctor? All questions from the last week that my trusty notepad has answered. I've found that a brief or abbreviated note is utterly useless to me because the chances of me remembering what that means are minimal. I find I have to write long-winded essays but at least I understand what I've written as a script and can apply the knowledge as I need to. Handy for knowing I've paid the bills in time and explaining what I need from the medical world or even being in the right place at the right time.

Numbness. Six months after my initial Covid infection, I noticed that my hands would suddenly let go of whatever I was holding unbidden by me. Not a huge drama if it was a letter but very annoying if it was a vase. This was followed by not being able to pick whatever had dropped back up because there was little or no sensation in my fingers. I ended up holding teapots between my palms to pour and performing other strange manoeuvres to function with numb hands. It's still happening and is still under investigation.

Neurologist - not interested, not his department apparently. The consultant physiotherapist was far more understanding and genuinely wanted to solve the problem, even being kind enough to refer me to a private open MRI scanner to help with my phobia. The result of that was a referral to a neurosurgeon to look at the newly grown bone in my neck that was potentially pressing on my spinal cord. In his wisdom, said surgeon gave me a phone call appointment because why would he want to actually look at the problem and give me a physical examination? That call was followed by - wait for it - a referral to physiotherapy! The physios asked me why I was back with them when it was the neurosurgeons I needed to see and referred me back to them again. An actual physical face to face appointment with a neurosurgeon happened. The result? Well, it's intermittent so you need to be referred by to neurology! And so the circle continues, bouncing back and forth between the three with no resolution.

I still have the numbness and dropping things going on. I daren't pick up my grandbabies for fear of dropping them and I feel terrible every time they want to be picked up and all I can do is sit down and kind of drag them towards me, all because of numbness in my hands. As I continue on the three point triangle of neurologist, physio, neurosurgeon, nothing improves and no answer seems in sight. Try getting holiday insurance with this going on!

But what has this to do with LC? Well, maybe nothing but the hyperacceleration identified by the rheumatologist of the arthritis in my joints makes me wonder about this new bone growth. Yet another gift from LC? Yes, I believe it is. Also, taking into account the well documented sensory changes attributed to LC, I believe it is the cause behind these changes in my body. *The Long Covid self-help guide* identifies that sensory changes can include numbness in the fingers and they have seen a lot of LC patients. In the meantime, as ever, I wait for the bouncing between hospital departments to resolve and maybe one day, I'll be able to pick up my grandchildren. Hope is all I have and some days, I find it to be in very short supply.

<u>O is for...</u>

Obesity. "Covid don't like fatties," one of the stars of Gogglebox said and it's true.
Being morbidly obese myself, I am always grateful that I was not bad enough with
any of my bouts of Covid to have been hospitalised but it has brought home some
grim realisations about the state of my health due to overeating and lack of exercise.
The fatigue brought on by LC means that exercise has to be thought about and
planned carefully. Food, my emotional crutch, has to be planned carefully but on
days where I can't laugh about it and on days where the frustration boils over, the
careful plans fly out of the window and the obscene amounts of unhealthy food are
once again part of my repertoire.

I'm not sure there is an answer or, at least not a simple answer, to this. Over
50 years of bad diet and lack of movement are not solved overnight, although the
desire to do anything to alleviate LC does help a little. It's more a need to finally start
resolving the emotional issues that make me overeat that will perhaps get me
started. And the decision not to beat myself up every time I overindulge or eat
nutritionally unsound food helps too. It's a very, very slow way forward and, if I could
afford it, maybe psychiatric or psychological appointments would help.

Of course, I wonder if I would even have LC if I had not been obese when I
caught Covid. Looking at my fellow LC sufferers in classes or at meetings makes
me feel a little better, in that we come in a variety of shapes and sizes so it is not a
given that obesity equals LC. However, I am sure it hasn't helped and, even though
I lapse on an almost daily basis, I really want to get healthier. I say healthier rather
than slim or thin because, for me, that's setting an unrealistic goal. But if I can
introduce healthier eating habits and get to a minimum of 3,000 steps a day (yes,
pathetic, isn't it?!) then it can only be good for my overall wellbeing.

There are support programmes out there and, when I hit the pre-diabetic, high
blood pressure and morbid obesity stage of my life, the GP referred me to a 12 week
programme funded by the NHS because I had become eligible to participate. It's a
good thing because it makes me look at my habits and examine my motivations. Will
power is key, as is the desire for change. I don't know if I will make the transition
down from morbidly obese to just obese or even lower, but it's a small sliver of hope

that if I lose weight, LC and subsequent Covid infections may not have as much devastating impact upon me and those around me each time.

Overwhelmed. Pre-LC, I'd get overwhelmed eventually by work, family life, health and so on after a long build up. A day of tears and shouting would sort it out in the main. Nowadays, I get overwhelmed by spending an hour doing a jigsaw puzzle! My brain literally shuts down and I get tearful, stressed and start hyperventilating because I feel I can't carry on or understand or do something. It's not as well defined as a full blown panic attack but it's like a switch in my brain pulling down the shutters and saying, "I can't, I can't, I can't," until my body produces a full on stress response. It brings anxiety, palpitations, tears, shaking and even nausea. Even when I use calming techniques, the feeling is overpowering and brings everything to a complete halt. It happens when I've been trying to concentrate for too long or doing too much physical activity or being emotionally battered. Every time.

What are the triggers for me? It can be anything. Trying to do a jigsaw, being in a group and trying to hold a conversation, a long walk, a medical appointment, housework, emotional overload, reading an email, getting out of bed and writing this book are all examples just from this week. It's too random to predict an exact activity that can set it off but, for me, it seems to be a prolonged (more than 20 minutes!) time of doing the same thing. It sort of goes back to my lack of attention span since LC but it's bigger and scarier than that. It's an all consuming feeling of panic, despair and incapability that shuts down all but the basic life support in my body.

Sometimes, I know it's coming and stop what I am doing and it recedes after an hour or two of mindless TV or sitting staring at the wall. Sometimes, it overpowers me and I just have to go to my room and lie crying in bed until I either fall asleep or calm down enough to have 'reset' myself. Even then, I can't seem to go back to what started the sensation of being overwhelmed that day. I have to have a complete break from that activity until the following day at the earliest. If I don't switch direction and instead go back to whatever triggered me, I find I can't complete what I was doing and start the whole feeling overwhelmed cycle again.

What's the answer? I have no idea other than to take a break if I feel the whole shutdown starting or stop what I'm doing when the feelings of being overwhelmed take over. Living life in small bite size chunks seems to be the way forward for now. That's why this book is in the format it is. If I'm lucky, I can get one word/definition written up in a day. It's taken it's time but you can see that I made it in the end!

Oximeter. When I was exceptionally breathless, I found an oximeter helped me keep an eye on my oxygen saturation levels as well as what felt like a racing heartbeat. It was quite cheap to buy online but I believe they are available in chemists as well. Because it just sits on the end of my finger, it doesn't feel in any way invasive or restrictive. That worked positively in two ways for me. When my readings were good, I was reassured that I was getting enough oxygen, despite being breathless. When the levels hit the more concerning levels, I could see when I needed to get medical help. Ideal oxygen saturation is between 96% and 100% but that is a very general guide so it was worth me finding out from my GP what was 'normal' for me so that I could keep an eye on my stats and not worry about what I should be at. There's a very good guidance chart at https://www.ridgmountpractice.nhs.uk/pulse-oximeters but again, it's only a guide to work from and it's a good idea to establish what is a usual personal rate before worrying that your readings are way off the guidance chart.

What I found interesting is that my 'normal' readings of oxygen saturation levels have dropped with each Covid infection. Pre-Covid, I was at 98% to 100% all the time. After the first (delta) infection, I'd dropped to 96% to 99%, which is still ok. After the second (omicron) infection, I was down to 95% to 97%. After the third (who knows? So many variants now!) infection, my new 'normal' is 94% to 97%. I see nothing disastrous in those readings but it is really interesting to see how my saturation levels have dropped and I wonder what will happen with each subsequent Covid infection that I get.

A quick note at the end of this part to say if there is no reading on the oximeter, get your fingers warm and it will work. Apparently, cold fingertips can't send out readings for the oximeter to pick up. Just a top tip, so you don't panic that it's broken. Unlike me, who was constantly sending them back because they 'didn't work' or thinking I must be far too ill to get a reading! D'oh!!

<u>P is for...</u>

Pacing. Pacing was something the rehab psychologists kept mentioning in our sessions. In all honesty, I didn't really grasp what they meant and got it all tangled up in my head with baseline, post exertional malaise, cost-benefit and listening to your body. I got very frustrated with myself every time I tried to live my life in the way I had pre-Covid and invariably ended up wiped out for the rest of the week. This led to a lot of self-recrimination and guilt, making it difficult to plan anything that didn't revolve around me and my needs. Wicked uncle guilt took over as my driving force because I didn't want my LC situation to be detrimental to those I love. That was a very low point in my LC life that still comes to haunt me if I'm not careful. It made me not want to carry on and inflict my illness upon others. It took a lot of time and mental anguish to get to the point of trying to adapt to a new way of thinking and living.

As I started to get to grips with finally beginning to understand about setting baselines and recognising my body's desperate red flag signals to me, I began to understand what pacing is and why I should bother with it. Hands up, it took me over a year to get this far (good old brain fog!) but now I feel that I comprehend what the idea behind pacing is, even if I still get it wrong sometimes.

Pacing is actually a simple concept. I need to work out how much is my absolute maximum energy level for the day and make sure I stay under that bar. By doing that, I can achieve more of the things I want/need to get done over the course of a week, rather than crash and burn after one day at full tilt. If I don't try and pace myself, the inevitable crash arrives, rendering me incapable for days on end. If I ignore my old instincts and ways of doing things, sometimes I still get it wrong but sometimes I get it right and can manage a week without a major crash.

That's not to say it's easy to get the pacing right. Even with the best planning, it can still go wrong because real life gets in the way and outside influences can also come in to play. But when I get a choice, I try to pace my day to ensure I can work within the level which means I can get up the next day and do other things. An example recently where I got it right was when I went to an exhibition, involving a train ride and a reasonably short walk to the exhibition centre. When I got there, I sat down and had a cup of tea because I knew I'd left enough time to be able to do so. Even the effort of sitting on a train for 40 minutes and walking perhaps 10 minutes more had taken its toll and I knew I couldn't enjoy what I had come to see. I'd paced it right! After about 45 minutes, I went into the exhibition and loved it and loved being able to do it and appreciate it. Coming out, again I had to sit and rest for another half hour before the trip back to the train station. Previously, I would have been raring to go for a meal and then on to another site, shop etc to make the most of the day and area.

By pacing myself, my recovery time from the exertion was less. I slept for a few hours after I arrived home but was actually recovered enough to cook a meal in the evening, which showed me a lot of progress, both physically and mentally. The family was divided - one was very supportive and went along with my pace happily, the other was the usual rolling eyes and 'You're going to bed again, then?' comment. That's family life and I am trying to focus on the more positive influences, although it can be tough and almost psychologically painful when guilt comes calling. However, as a pacing exercise, I felt good about it and logged it mentally as an achievement because I knew I hadn't gone too mad and tried to live my old life, which would have had far more familial impact over the following days. I was lethargic for the following two days but capable of functioning at baseline level, so that told me I am on the road to pacing my new life! I still have a long way to go before I get it right more times than I get it wrong but I feel that I am finally on the pathway. It's yet another case of keep plugging away at it and I may get there in the end.

Pain. And the perception of pain. Two P's for the price of one. I was always a bit of a wimp with pain but could try and hold it in a lot of the time. For example, I could make it through a six hour tattoo session but a toothache had me crying like a baby. Since Covid, my resistance to pain has dropped to the toothache level for everything. A small knock against a counter or stubbing my toe has my pain receptors screaming at me and, more often than not, a sudden unwelcome burst of tears pouring down my face, which doesn't help with the family's tolerance levels. The 'Again?' expressions cross their faces, no matter how briefly.

I can't explain whether it is my brain deludedly telling me I am feeling more pain in everything or whether it is a genuine increase in the level of pain or lowering of pain tolerance. I don't want to use the Buprenorphine patches that I have been prescribed because I don't want to add addiction to everything else that LC has gifted me. But when you wake up every day with most things aching, then increase the pain level from the smallest 'injury' or headache, back ache, muscle spasm by at least 50% of what it used to be, it's tempting. And I use them sometimes because I need to function. I need to carry on.

The constant pain and increased perception of it makes me tired, which adds to the fatigue, creating a perpetual cycle that cannot be ignored. It can't be cured (at the moment!) so it has to be managed. I can't say I'm managing it well but some days, the pain can be managed. Blotted out even sometimes. But then the next day starts up with the aching head, aching joints and it's back on the merry go round again. Managing it or living with it? Not too much difference when the pain comes calling.

Palpitations. It was after the third bout of Covid that I started to get some very scary palpitations that made me think that a heart attack was imminent. A holter monitor showed that they were actually happening and it wasn't just my imagination. Hallelujah! A test that actually showed positive results rather than the usual negatives. They weren't damaging my heart and there were no other heart issues showing. But the palpitations carried on for a long time after the Covid infection then suddenly vanished as if they had never been there. According to various online articles, heart issues are a big part of Covid so I guess it's logical that they form a part of Long Covid too. I'm lucky that the palpitations have receded for me but that doesn't stop the occasional uh-oh from me every time the odd thump and skip happens. Making notes of when they recur has made me realise that they are now only triggered by high stress levels, rather than being a daily occurrence. To deal with the stress is to deal with the palpitations. So simple in print and almost impossible in real life!

PASC (post acute sequelae SARS Cov 2 infection). Yet another way of saying Long Covid. It's a bit of a mouthful whichever way you look at it and saying "I have PASC" to medics and civilians alike meets with a blank look in the eyes, recognition only dawning when you say, "Long Covid". Although it's more official sounding than either Long Covid or Post Covid Syndrome, I feel this definition/diagnosis is going to be short lived in the media.

Patterns. Quite early on in the LC journey, I was told to try to identify patterns because that would make pacing easier. LC is so unpredictable that any pattern other than fatigue after every activity can be exceptionally difficult to spot. Imagine how I felt after 19 months of LC when I finally spotted a pattern! If I have an exhausting day due to travelling or a lot of brain work, two days later, I absolutely tank on the physical and mental energy. Every time. I take that to be a pattern. Being able to predict the pattern theoretically makes it easier to pace and plan around it. If I plan a down day for 'day 3' and quiet days for the following two days, the days after that allow a gradual recharge of my energy bank. If I try to push through 'day 3', it inevitably ends in a complete crash with days and even weeks of Zombie days following unrelentingly. It's not always easy to plan but I have found that the pattern brings a small window of predictability to the unpredictable and can help manage the unmanageable.

Unless of course, the pattern breaks down. I was too confident in my day 3 system and coached about 100 miles, stayed away 5 days, coached back, went up and down to London by train for two days in a row, then drove about 100 miles, stayed away for five days and drove back again. I had applied the day 3 rest principle so all was good, wasn't it? I spent the fortnight after this extreme exertion in and out of bed with practically zero mental capacity, not much ability to communicate and an absolutely ravenous desire to consume as much sugar and carbohydrate as possible to build up even false energy levels. Two weeks after that and I was still feeling the effects. With hindsight, it was way, way too much to attempt in such a condensed period of time and even the day 3 pattern rest plan came crashing down. My conclusion is that the patterns hold good when circumstances are 'normal' and there are no major changes outside of what passes for normality. When life throws a spanner into these plans, though, even the best thought out plans and patterns have to be rethought.

Post Covid Syndrome. Post Covid SYndrome is a relabelling of Long Covid to make it more believable to society and certain members of the medical profession. Yes, Long Covid and Post Covid Syndrome are one and the same thing. Long Covid is a thing but so many folk think it means you still have Covid or, as mentioned above, they think it's a tool for swinging the lead and doesn't really exist. But to have a syndrome - well, that's a game changer! I must have a long term health condition if I have a syndrome! And it must be a real thing if it's a syndrome. Sigh.

Post Exertional Malaise. It's not the same as being tired after exercising or being busy all day. It's not even the fatigue after a build up of not listening to my body's cues. Post Exertional Malaise hits me a couple of days after a big expenditure of energy, be that mental, emotional or physical and it's like being hit by a truck. Like the fatigue, all of a sudden, movement, speech and thought are all impossible and the only thing that is possible is to lie down. It's also not a case that a quick rest can restore energy levels. It can take days or even weeks to get back up to the new normal energy levels with me being able to do nothing other than quietly observe the recuperation almost from outside of my own body and mind.

When I first heard the term, the word Malaise was the part that stuck with me. I'd always associated the term with laziness, hypochondria and general lead-swinging malingering. I'm sure I'm not alone in that. I first heard the term in the post Covid rehab group and my initial reaction was that we were being called lazy malingerers. However, the more I read about it (mainly in *The Long Covid self-help guide*), the more I understood what happened to me the two or three days after a massive energy expending day/hour/time and why it didn't happen the day after. It's a build up of energy draining that goes hand in hand with the fatigue, so just being active the day after drains the reserves further, leading to a crash with PEM.

The weirdest thing about PEM is that sometimes, it is so out of proportion to the amount of activity I have done. Just the other day, I had done a mere 500 steps and had a generally quiet, recovering time then I was hit with PEM and fatigue two days later. I couldn't understand why until I thought about what had gone on during my quiet day. I had heard that a friend had died and had been speaking to her niece about the funeral arrangements. It then occurred to me that, physically, I had done little but the emotional expenditure that day had been huge. In turn, this led me to thinking about the time I did a jigsaw, concentrating on it for hours, and two days later, PEM kicked in. My conclusion is that post exertional does not just refer to the physical side of exertion, it's mental and emotional exertion as well. Wow. That's an all rounder that makes life just that bit tougher to navigate.

I have had to come to accept that sometimes, it is just unavoidable. With some serious pre-planning, it can be avoided with judiciously spaced exertion, rest and so on. For example, I planned a day of doing minimal activity and no going out after a post Covid rehab exercise class, thereby avoiding a huge fatigue crash. Another time, it just wasn't possible so the inevitable PEM set in two days later. In itself, that can be catered for in terms of calendar planning but what is impossible to judge is how long it will take to regain the energy I have lost. Occasionally, I am lucky and it only lasts two days. Another time, it can be a week. Mental exertion is harder to plan for and as for emotional exertion, how on earth can you plan for that? For me, PEM is helpfully predictable and unhelpfully unpredictable and yet another part of LC that I have to manage that affects those around me too.

<u>Q is for...</u>

Questions. So many questions and so few answers - that is the ongoing issue with LC in terms of research, help available and day to day life. I guess that's how it is with all new illnesses, viruses and disabilities. Every LCer has questions and even if some answers are forthcoming, the questions increase with each day. For me, the biggest question is, "Will this ever go away?" closely followed by, "Will I ever feel completely well again?" At this moment of time, both are unanswerable, which brings me to how answerable questions really are or can be in terms of LC.

LC is a new thing. No one has all the answers - or even many of the answers - and it is too new to have its own consultants and dedicated hospital departments. There are services dedicated to LC, cobbled together from chronic fatigue, physiotherapy, neurology and so on but no dedicated departments. The mimicry that LC specialises in has us LCers chasing round a variety of hospital departments to try to explain our symptoms and often, through no fault of their own or our own, the wrong questions are being asked by the specialists in those fields because LC is so very tricky. Because the wrong questions are being asked, LC doesn't provide answers to standard tests. The questions often remain unanswered, the patient is discharged from that department with no resolution and the merry-go-round goes on.

How can the right questions be asked? An almost impossible question to answer. I think the key is two-fold. If more research directly with LC patients is promoted and the results of LCer surveys etc become higher profile, the medical community may be able to catch up, develop LC specialisms and more answers may be forthcoming. One of the biggest barriers to this is the potentially transient nature of LC. Where some LCers have recovered, the argument is that it is a temporary illness so valuable resources and training should not be wasted on something that is impermanent. Those of us approaching and marking three year anniversaries would beg to differ, arguing that even if a miracle occurs and LC suddenly vanishes, so much of our body has changed irrevocably or been so damaged by LC that something permanent needs to happen in the medical community and in wider society to ensure that the best care is available and as many questions as possible are answered.

 is a group of LCers with a scientific background who are generating patient led hypotheses and scientific papers to try and push the research further, based on LC experiences. The point of interest in this is that LC patients are banding together to try to be heard and a lot of the hypotheses are very interesting. There are others out there - some real, some fake and some just trying to part you with your money. Never sign up for anything that wants a paid subscription until you are 100% sure of the motivation and genuine status would be my advice!

There comes a point of frustration where questions arise far more than answers and, as an unheard LCer, you feel like giving up on the system and taking your chances with the quacks and the moneymakers out there. It's understandable and shows how desperate some of us are to feel well and capable again. It really is up to the scientists to push forward and use LCers who are desperate to help to discover more about the illness. Research and study is the way to start answering the LC questions. If the funding can happen, hopefully the studies and results will be forthcoming. When/if it is, let's hope the questions can be answered.

<u>R is for...</u>

Recovery. "Is this ever going away? Will I ever get better?" are words I use most days, along with many LCers I have spoken to. Rehab clinics tell us to stop thinking like this and accept that the changes LC has made to us could well be permanent. It's an easy thing to say and very difficult to do. Where so much is still unknown about LC, there is no way of knowing if everyone can make a full recovery. Some people have - at the time of writing, many of those who have recovered had the Omicron strain but others have recovered too, which gives those of us with original, Alpha and Delta strains hope. But maybe it's time for me to stop thinking about recovery as a return to pre-Covid health and ways. Maybe I need to think of any improvement as a recovery rather than a step towards it.

If I look back to where I was when I first had LC, I can see improvements. On a non fatigue day, I can walk a lot further, concentrate more and hold a conversation for longer than the first days, weeks and months with LC. What is frustrating is that on a fatigue day, these achievements are almost all wiped out. However, using the dreaded journaling tool, I have been able to see some very small steps towards improvement and recovery. The zombie days, the crashes and so on can sometimes be more manageable because I am more aware of the patterns that activity and rest demonstrate. Obviously, there's times when my LC is just as bad as at the beginning, which brings despair blanketing down upon me. However, on average, there is a general movement upwards on my baseline of how each part of LC affects me.

Can I look at this as recovery? It's a case of having to change my mindset about what recovery is and what I can reasonably expect. When nothing is certain or known, it's hard to know what to expect and that's where talking to other LCers is so valuable. Not to set up some sort of league table as to who is making the most progress, who is fully recovered etc but just to talk through the times when recovery looks as if it is complete fantasy and to celebrate the small improvements that are steps along the way. It could be that where I am now is as good as I am ever going to get but I don't think that should make me stop trying to get better than I am right now.

I feel I must use any tool I can find to keep the improvements coming or, if they have plateaued, at least to stop from going backwards again. That can be exercise, mental 'brain training' apps, breathing exercises, meditation - the list is ongoing and added to regularly. I also need to stop feeling guilty about taking the time to try and heal myself as that is a huge block in my recovery. Allow myself to believe I can recover and I am allowed to take the necessary time and make the necessary effort to try to make recovery happen, even if it means I have to stop helping others for the time that it takes for me to do the daily routines. Mental recovery and rehab is just as important as losing weight and improving my lung capacity and general fitness.

Recovery feels like a dream that is far, far away but it is a goal, perhaps unrealistic but until more is known, it has to exist in hope. Taking each movement on the baseline as a step forward, even if it is a long time coming, I can hope for that recovery to a level where life is worth living again. Maybe I will never recover fully to where I used to be but if I can make enough progress to get to the point of life not being torture and something I actually enjoy again, well, that will be a recovery for me.

Rehab. After the first wave of Covid in 2020, the UK government set up clinics to offer rehab to survivors of Covid-19 and LCers. Regional centres were set up in England, some being more successful than others. Some clinics were led by doctors from a variety of specialisms, such as cardiology, respiratory specialisms, rheumatology, neurology and so on. Others are run by psychologists and physiotherapists. Success rates seem to vary according to which area of expertise runs the centre. https://www.england.nhs.uk/2020/10/nhs-to-offer-long-covid-help/ lists the ideals for each centre and the thinking behind the creation of the centres. They are to get us better! The Oxford clinic has produced a very helpful book *The Long Covid Self Help Guide* as a result of their interactions with patients and it shows in the reading of the book.

Sadly, where LC is such an unknown and the NHS is so understaffed, a lot of the clinics fall a long way short of the ideals set out in 2020. The way to get referred is to ask your GP and, if they decide you are exhibiting symptoms of LC, they may refer you to your nearest rehab clinic. My experiences with my local rehab clinic varied wildly. My initial assessment followed the standard guidelines and was carried out by a physiotherapist who offered me a six week psychology course on Zoom with a group of other LCers to be followed by exercise sessions. At that stage, I couldn't string two words together coherently and just getting to the assessment appointment was an achievement.

The Zoom class was disappointing to say the least. Ten strangers were thrust together with nothing in common other than the fact that they had Long Covid and their experiences and symptoms were wildly different. The psychologists running the course insisted everyone had their cameras on all the time, which was intimidating for many of us. There followed a two hour lecture each fortnight, which I didn't have the brain function to maintain concentration for, so much was lost on me. Halfway through the course, we all had an opportunity for a half hour one to one interaction with the psychologist. That was the highlight for me, as the rest of it was just too overwhelming. I feel that it would have been far more productive to have had those individual half hour sessions more regularly than the two hour group where people said very little. I guess time constraints make that impossible but I did come away from the course feeling that there were 12 hours of my life I wouldn't see again and those 12 hours could have been better used sleeping! Chatting post course to some of my fellow Zoomers, we agreed it could have been far better managed to suit LC and the ignoring of the lack of ability to concentrate was a real obstacle to feeling a sense of help and achievement.

A fellow LCer who was referred to a different clinic was told by the psychologist to work less and stop talking about LC and get back to normality. After two sessions! She was then discharged because there was nothing else they could do and she should be proud of her recovery. Recovery? She still has LC and I'm not sure that any recovery could be measured after two weeks of sessions. Hearing this, I suddenly felt very blessed to have had my twelve hours of boredom and frustration. At least I had gained a few bits of knowledge from it, although it was not until I read the Oxford clinic's book that I actually understood what they meant. The greatest benefit I gained from the group sessions was when a small number of us set up our own WhatsApp group. I have spoken to and shared so much since we set that up and had felt reassurance, understanding and love from everyone in it.

The exercise classes filled me with horror. I was unfit before Covid hit so the thought of enforced exercise was traumatic. The classes were run by physios and it depended who was taking the class as to how much use they were. There was a standard set of exercises that all the patients were supposed to do, irrespective of ability, symptoms etc. A few of the physios made us all feel like they had drawn the short straw and had to be with the LC malingerers and so their objective was to push everyone beyond their abilities, apart from the class favourite, because they were just not interested in finding out what individual capabilities were. On my first day, the physio just shouted to the room, "Right, warm up as usual." I just stood there, thinking he may come and explain something or maybe give an introduction. No chance. I had to ask one of the other participants what to do. You get the picture.

However, one of the physios was magnificent and made a huge difference to my attitude towards the classes with his approach. He understood that we were all at different stages of LC and had different abilities (or lack thereof in my case!) and tailored his class to suit the eight individuals in it, welcoming everyone in as they arrived and asking if there were any new symptoms or things he should be aware of. I was exhausted afterwards and the post exertional malaise set in but I found, as the six weeks went on, my recovery time was faster. I was offered a second set and accepted the online classes with this man. Never have I felt so positive after exercising and I did feel that my stamina had improved. He even went and bought himself a copy of the Oxford clinic's book so that he could better understand his patients. I would love to name him so he can receive some well deserved kudos but I feel it could make life more difficult for him amongst his peers if I did.

The drawback to LC rehab was that, as soon as you had been registered with the service for a year and/or done the online psychology and exercise classes, you were discharged. My LC WhatsApp group all said the same thing. "But we still have Long Covid! What are we supposed to do now?" The answer was more or less to just get on with it, going back to the misguided theory that LC clears up after a year. Once again, we are cast into the void of LC. Because it is still being researched, because the NHS has a lack of staff, because LC is so wide ranging no individual specialist can deal with it, we just have to crack on and make our own way through it after the year with the rehab service. Maybe it's different at other clinics? I can't say. It's certainly worth going for the rehab classes if offered them and they do offer health benefits but it does come as a crashing disappointment to be discharged knowing the initial problem for which you were referred is still ongoing with no sign of disappearing any time soon and no more help will be forthcoming.

In *The Long Covid Handbook*, the advice at the end that has been specifically written for GPs warns them to be aware of 'therapist only' run services. The dangers are not screening for Post Exertional Malaise, using exercise as therapy and CBT, as none of these are LC specific, which is obviously what is needed in our cases. The whole spiel I have written above maybe underlines the reasons why this is the case. I'm going to wager that the majority of UK GPs will not have read Medinger and Altmann's book and therefore not be aware of this advice. They may or may not be open to being informed about it but I would wager that limited NHS resources are going to mean that anyone with the therapist led services near them have no chance of getting referred to a specialist centre such as the one at Oxford. Postcode lottery, indeed.

Reinfection. It's always lurking at the back of my mind - what if I get Covid again? Will this be it? Again, because so little is known about Covid and LC, I have been told completely opposing 'facts' about a reinfection. The first is along the lines of 'don't worry, it won't be as bad as the first time'; the second is similar to the first plus 'it'll make no difference to your LC'; the third is similar to the first but with a worrying 'of course, your LC will get much worse'; and the fourth? That's the pants scaring one. 'A reinfection could kill you'. Based on those pieces of advice, I should either live in an hermetically sealed apartment for the rest of my days or I should be out and about and partying like it's 1999. Kind of makes the whole advice thing a bit pointless, doesn't it?

On to my experience of reinfection now. My first reinfection was horrible and many symptoms were the same as before - the headache, the inability to get warm, the cough etc. - but I had new aftereffects added to my LC that I still haven't been able to shake, like the pain in every joint. On the whole, being Omicron, I would say it was milder than the first time but the aftereffects are a lot more painful. My second reinfection was the scariest of all three because it felt like I was drowning every time I was at less than a 90 degree angle and definitely when I lay down. The main symptoms like the headache and cough were a lot milder but the flooding of the lungs was a very new and very unwelcome addition to my overall collection. Luckily, the fluid seemed to clear up after a few weeks, although I have more of a permanent cough than before. My LC group have had a variety of reinfection experiences from quite mild and hardly noticeable symptoms to a full scale month in intensive care!

I think it's reasonable to say that reinfection adds to the ongoing LC symptoms, although it doesn't necessarily make the LC itself worse. This leaves me and other LCers with the choice of totally isolating ourselves from the world forever (or at least until LC has gone!) or getting out there, with or without masks, and doing what we can with our remaining time, living as full a life as we have left to us with LC. There's no right or wrong answer and the answer you choose changes daily. Reinfection is undoubtedly a huge threat to my health but so is living in isolation forever. It's something to be pondered at length.

Research. There's plenty of official medical research going on and a variety of medical trials, in which we are invited to participate but only if you live in a certain area and can do certain things. However, the most important, self-empowering research I have found is my own. I don't mean that in an 'I know better than the professionals' way because, in the case of drugs, tests, scans etc, I really don't and I'm not qualified to or capable of carrying out scientific research projects. But I know my own body better than anyone else can. Because LC symptoms are so varied from person to person, it can be very hit and miss with what is being researched medically and even whether the symptoms are being attributed to LC or not.

With the brain fog and fatigue, prolonged periods of study and concentration are impossible for me right now. How I deal with it is by being in groups of fellow LCers and having the ever-present Google to hand, along with my trusty notebook and pen. When I find someone else has the same symptoms or even if they don't, I'm straight on to Google, looking for books, articles and so on. This has led to some wild experiments (we won't even talk about my collagen pills experiment to help my joints!) but also some successes like the ginger and turmeric gummies for inflammation. I'm not advocating being irresponsible with your own health by trying insane stuff or spending money on 'miracle' cures that are fake. I look at my symptoms and try to find a possible cause (eg sudden rise in blood pressure - could that be a mega salt intake over the last few days or could it be caused by LC and the dysautonomia? The key is to find what else could be causing symptoms before automatically ascribing the blame to LC). Once I have a cause, I try to look for potential solutions or treatments. Sometimes, things are easy to try at home like the omega 3 supplements but it's always worth checking with a GP before embarking on even a self prescribed treatment, as I found out the hard way.

Arming myself with my research and my notes, I have been able to present a reasonably coherent argument to my GP or the hospital specialist that outline my symptoms and why I think they are LC related. If appropriate, I ask about a course of treatment that I can either self-administer or ask them to prescribe and so on. That's not to say I am always listened to or helped. Far from it. But by going in armed with my own research, I feel I'm giving myself the best shot at getting help from the professionals. If it doesn't happen, well, that person was never going to help me but it's worth going in with every discovery to lay out before them. You never know.

Resignation. Nowhere near acceptance but one step up from anger is the best way I can describe how I understand resignation to be. Acceptance is more positive, resignation is more negative. "I have LC and it's always going to be like this," is a very frequent thought that goes through my mind, along with, "It's here forever so I may as well get used to being stuck like this." It's a step up to accepting my fate but is far more negative and depressing than being positive and looking forward. It can be the wallowing in self pity day or it can be the 'my future is over' day or it can be the 'I have no control over this' day or the 'I'm ruining my family's lives with this,' day. It feels hopeless and terrifying and very passive. LC is being done to me, not me taking hold of what I have. It's not always possible to be upbeat and that's when the resignation to a life changing illness? disease? disability? comes in. It's a state marked by depression and anxiety. Not a good place to be. When people say, "You're resigned to your fate," I don't think they realise just how much they are condemning you to a future lacking in hope with those words. Resignation is natural and fine as an intermediate stage towards acceptance but really isn't a place to want to dwell for long.

Rest. Before LC, I had thought of rest as lying on the bed either nodding off to sleep or being quiet with a book or some music. I thought that a quick rest would refresh me and bring my energy levels back to 'normal' and, more often than not, it used to. Since Covid-19, my energy banks are depleted and don't refill with a rest alone, although it is essential to stop when my body/mind tells me to. Through talking to other LCers and psychologists, I have come to realise that rest is not sleep and there are many forms of rest, with each being vital to be able to maximise the chances of having a good LC day.

Dr Saundra Dalton-Smith in her 2018 book, *Sacred Rest: Recover your Life, Renew your Energy, Restore your Sanity* identifies seven types of rest (not sleep, that's a different thing) to enable individuals to achieve their maximum recovery and potential. She identifies physical, mental, spiritual, emotional, sensory, social and creative rest areas that need to have attention paid to them. I am only in a position to comment on rest areas that I personally have experienced with LC and give my definition or understanding of what that means for me. Again, I am thinking personally and am in no position to offer advice or guidance for others and am not seeking to actively promote or denigrate her work.

There is emotional rest - that time when you need to take a break from all the emotions surrounding you, not just the LC emotions but the ones arising from family, friends, work etc. Far easier said than done, but breathing exercises help with the emotional rest because I am so focussed on counting breaths that I forget to think about what is bothering me. Dr Boon Lim has a breathing exercise on YouTube that helps lower the heart rate, potentially reset the autonomic system and provide a sort of rest. The emotional rest kind of marries up well with Dr D-S's identification of social rest too, I have found. If I take a social break, quite often my emotions calm down and I don't feel so inflamed about everything.

The physical rest is, for me, what it says it is - a break from physical activity, preferably in a prone position and with no stimulation, not even a book or calming music. It is a state of total calm and nothingness. Some people find yoga, meditation or breathing exercises help achieve this state. Let's say I'm still working on this one. Mental rest is another thing. Taking a break from intense mental activity hasn't been a problem for me. I can veg out in front of the TV or sit gazing aimlessly at a wall with no difficulty. It's maintaining any kind of mental activity that I find difficult. An LCer I spoke to needed to calm it down but not completely switch off because she was working. What seemed to work for her was doing a 'lower grade' mental activity such as colouring or a children's puzzle.

Sensory rest is another big area for me. I can get very overwhelmed with sounds, conversations in a room full of people and even watching the latest blockbuster at the cinema can leave me feeling exhausted. I have found my best way for sensory rest is very similar to others - calming breathing, shutting my eyes, covering my ears and generally trying to shut off as many senses as I can calms my overheated senses and being alone in a room (even the bathroom) again overlaps with the social rest aspect.

Whatever the LC truth for people, rest is a very individual thing and is actually nothing to do with sleep. I may go so far as to say that rest is more important to me than sleep because it helps refill my energy tanks - never completely full but even a 1% increase is greeted with my gratitude and delight.

<u>S is for...</u>

Self Help. A phrase I have used to those I have had contact with over the decades is, "You have to be proactive, not reactive." It's a motto I have tried to live by, although not always successfully if I am honest. One thing that LC has taught me is the need for proactivity in everything. Where Covid is such a new thing, every discovery around it is also new. Information is not disseminated fast enough or widely enough for help with LC. Even the 'specialists' in LC treatment, rehab or whatever you want to call it don't know it all. As an LCer, I have been in the position too many times of trying to find out the Information and bring it to their attention. Sometimes, that has been met with appreciation, other times I have been made to feel like I am interfering and wasting time.

I have been combing the internet, borrowing library books etc to try and find out what I can do to help myself. Sometimes it's a supplement, sometimes it's an exercise, sometimes it's a failure and another, "Help me!" to my GP. It's exhausting mentally and emotionally, especially when I am trying to deal with the brain fog that means I can't understand or process what I am reading and the fatigue that means even half an hour of intense study results in a potential crash later on. But I won't stop because that would mean I have given up on myself and I'm not at that stage yet!

Self help is a huge part of LC acceptance too. By admitting I need to help myself, it has kind of led me into accepting the fact that I have to change and have to adapt to my new LC life. There are days where I don't want to help myself and I want someone else to take up the burden and just hand it all to me on a plate. Realistically, I know that only I can help myself, whether that's researching LC or doing the exercises prescribed to me, taking medication or whatever.

The self help mindset has to be at the heart of my recovery, acceptance and my LC life. Without it, there will be no inspiration to even try and get out of bed in the mornings and no chance of moving the baseline of living even one point higher. Accepting the bad days is easier when I know I am helping myself by taking those days as just a part of my life and refusing to just let LC and lassitude win.

Shaking. Or the shakes. A new warning system that my body has put into place when I have physically exerted myself way over the limit. Just as the hoarseness warns me that I have been too busy mentally or emotionally (sometimes physically), my hands start shaking uncontrollably when I have pushed the physical stuff too far. If I ignore the shakes and carry on, they travel down to my legs via my arms and torso. I end up looking like I am going cold turkey off drugs and there is absolutely nothing that can stop it apart from lying down to rest. Trying to take it as a positive, I'm looking at the shakes as a good warning sign that my body provides and one I should definitely listen to. As a negative, it can be really embarrassing to be sitting shaking all over on a bus or train but even that has a positive - people tend to offer me a seat and give me a wide berth at the same time!

Sleep. Specifically insomnia or lack of sleep. Being fatigued and having Post Exertional Malaise means you sleep a lot, right? I wish that were true! I feel the need to sleep most of the day on most days but the actual passing out into a state of altered consciousness? Not so much. I have fatigue and I have trouble sleeping. That's a sentence that makes no sense, like a lot of LC. Apparently, even LCers who spend 18 hours a day asleep spend their waking time feeling tired and fatigued, so long sleeps aren't an answer to fatigue either. Is there an answer? There are so many medical articles and books on sleep that it's far too big a subject to fit into a couple of paragraphs here. I want to touch on a few things that I have found have helped or information I have discovered that I would like to share.

The sleep I get is apparently non-restorative, meaning you can sleep for hours or minutes and the effect is the same. Little or no repair work is done by the body, rest just doesn't happen and a whole other host of nasties happen that result in - wait for it - fatigue and brain fog. It's more than a vicious cycle, it's a completely destructive cycle. LC gives us fatigue and brain fog and our bodies want to sleep to repair and recover but LC gives us non-restorative sleep that gives is brain fog and fatigue, that means we get non-restorative sleep, that means we get... and so on forever!

Are sleeping pills the answer? I can honestly say I turn to them when I have had a few days of less than 3 hours' sleep in total but an online article by Dr Daniel Kripke has made me more wary than ever about using them. I know that they can be addictive so have never used them for more than two nights in a row and that long term usage can lead to insomnia when you stop taking them because you are so used to them that the brain forgets how to sleep by itself. When I read articles on www.darksideofsleepingpills.com, I was shocked and horrified. Dr Kripke identifies alarming cancer and mortality rates in people who take even a maximum of 18 sleeping pills in a year and highlights respiratory problems as another side effect. It's incredibly sobering reading material but, in all honesty, I still take the odd one here and there because I am that desperate to sleep.

I use all the 'sleep hygiene' techniques cited in books, magazines and by TV health gurus. There are too many to get into here because it's such a huge, complex subject but I am talking, in general, about no heavy meals after 8pm, no blue light activity on phones or tablets at least 2 hours before bed, getting up after 20 minutes if the mind is racing, having the bedroom at an ambient temperature with no TV in the room and so on. The list is a lot longer and new suggestions are always popping up in magazines and newspaper articles. Sometimes they work for me, sometimes they don't so I can't comment on their efficacy or otherwise. Matthew Walker (a neuroscientist) has written a helpful book called *Why We Sleep* on the topic of sleep with many suggestions to help insomnia. Many other authors have written on the topic of sleep, dreaming and its benefits. As yet, there is nothing about LC and sleep, which is what I need. It's well worth reading a lot of different source material to get new ideas and techniques to try. Sleep and lack of restorative sleep is here to stay until a reason for why LC is affecting it so badly is found. Keep trying is the only advice I have.

Smell. As in sense of or lack thereof. I lost my sense of smell on the first day of Covid and it took 15 months to get to about 70% of where it was before. I've been through being able to smell nothing (more than a bit concerning when you have food allergies that smell helps to detect), through to everything smelling like faeces, regardless of what it was, through to cat litter smelling like flowers (guess who was on litter tray duty in this phase!!), through to being able to smell very strong smells very faintly. There is a medical term - parosmia - for a distorted sense of smell and it is being added to the symptoms of LC.

In December 2022, an article in The Times drew my attention and gave me some hope. https://www.thetimes.co.uk/article/loss-of-smell-in-long-covid-patients-caused-by-immune-response-say-scientists-htz0tvldm George Sandeman reported on a study by Duke University in the USA which found that loss of smell in people with Long Covid is caused by the damage to nerve cells in the nose by an immune response. At last, LC is being taken seriously in academic circles and studies being conclusive enough to be reported in national newspapers.

Apparently, LC patients have fewer nerve cells to detect smells, which could be down to the damage caused by the immune response to Covic, Long Covid etc. Now that such research has been done and conclusions drawn, maybe a treatment can be designed to help LC sufferers regain some of their previous ability. In the case of parosmia, the British Rhinological Society has a variety of suggestions, which are discussed in *The Long Covid self-help guide*. There are ways of training the brain to identify smells correctly again, which are not specific to LC sufferers but nonetheless valuable.

And if that can be done for the sense of smell, maybe LC will emerge as a condition to be taken seriously and be given resources to design treatments within already existing treatments for other conditions. It's a long way away but there's a glimmer of hope for now. Personally, I'm sad that the used cat litter smelling like flowers phase has gone but I'm grateful that my full sense of smell is still lacking when clearing the products of my cat's partying lifestyle!

Sneezing. Randomly, I now start to sneeze repeatedly without being able to stop for minutes at a time. It's only been since my first Covid infection and there's no obvious cause. Antihistamines and blowing the nose don't stop it. Then, just as randomly, it stops again. I can't say for sure it's an LC thing but it's only been happening since LC invaded so I suspect it to be the case. It's not harming my health but it can be quite tiring and is definitely very annoying for me and those who have to listen to the explosive, "A-whoooo-shoooo," every few seconds for about five minutes. In a theatre, at the dramatically paused moment of a scene, it can be exceptionally embarrassing too!

Stammer. A weird thing happened when chatting to the LC rehab group. One lady commented that she had started stammering since being diagnosed with LC. Then another person exclaimed, "Yes, so have I!" The following week, a couple more people said they had noticed it. Group hysteria maybe? No, actually. After the sessions had finished, I suddenly began to stammer. I kept a close note and found that it was whenever I was approaching the tired rather than fatigued state or when super stressed. It's become more pronounced as time has gone on. It's not incapacitating, thankfully and I use the Stop! Technique, as I do for panic and it calms it. If only certain people would understand that rolling their hands in the international 'get a move on gesture' while rolling their eyes really doesn't help and, in fact, only makes me stutter more because I'm trying to rush!

The neurologist was far too keen to get me off his books to even bother discussing it, even though I was stammering trying to tell him about the stammer! I was discharged with nothing coherent one way or another on whether a stammer is part of LC or not. For me, it seems too much of a coincidence that so many (I would estimate 70%) of the LC rehab group had developed it. Another area that needs research but with neurologists like the one I saw, it's not going to happen any time soon so managing it and adapting are the only options. I used the word stammer because that is the UK word but stutter - the USA version - applies equally.

Stop! A technique of sorts that I use to stop the racing thoughts, the panic and obsessing about LC. When the panic starts, I have to shout Stop! to myself, either out loud or in my head. Then I have to look for five different things and try to hear four different things, feel textures of three different things and repeat until the racing thoughts have stopped and I am breathing normally again. I'm sure there is a proper name for this technique - it is something I have cobbled together from reading various books on panic and overthinking - and I don't want to detract from its creators. I just don't know a proper name for it to be able to credit them. There are activities for taste and smell - one thing you can smell and two you can taste - but they are irrelevant to me at this stage of LC, as I have muted awareness in both of these senses. It's a very simple thing that can be done anywhere and it's definitely not a cure but it has got me through some tough situations like the dreaded MRI or hours and hours in A and E, along with mentally putting my David Bowie album collection into chronological release order, reverse chronological release order, alphabetical order... you get the idea!

Symptoms. Symptoms seem to be the thing that makes LC unbelievable to many non sufferers. Gez Medinger states there are over 205 identified LC symptoms so far. Where it's all so wide-ranging across so many people, I do have sympathy for the unbelievers. Personally, I have found that each bout of Covid-19 has brought new, additional symptoms with it, prompting a "You've got that as well now?" type incredulous response from relatives and medics alike. Understandable because I also think, "What, this too?" as I try to work out how to deal with the latest symptom for my collection.

The problem I have found with such a plethora of symptoms is that it's easy to brush off something potentially serious like the heart or blood pressure issues as being LC and ignore something potentially life-threatening. Conversely, it's been very easy for me to fall into the almost hypochondriac state of watching each new symptom like a fat puma waiting to pounce and drag it off to the GP. It's hard to know what to do and I'm now on first name terms with the GP's receptionists as a result. Medinger has a wonderful chart in his book *The Long Covid Handbook* that shows percentages of the most common symptoms and it's been such a help for me in trying to determine which route I should take between shrugging it off and getting it investigated. A fellow LCer had been paranoid about a rash that had appeared on his hands, fearing that Covid had damaged his liver. With the chart, it turns out skin rashes appear in around 12% of LCers, reassuring my friend enough to be able to get it checked out without being in fear of the results.

I believe the list of symptoms will keep growing as LC lasts longer and more is discovered. Some of the symptoms have treatments (not cures!) like the fatigue, the blood pressure and so on. My worry is that combining all the treatments could leave an imbalance that makes my body decide it doesn't want to play any more so I am probably over-cautious about accepting new treatments and trying new techniques for a new symptom until I have got a mental measure on what is happening with the current ones. I feel the whole symptoms category is a labyrinth to be negotiated carefully and one where the goal posts keep changing daily.

T is for...

Tachycardia. The racing heart rate came as part and parcel of my third Covid infection. Unlike the palpitations, it hasn't cleared up and gone but it has improved a bit. My heart still races and can be quite painful at times but, as there seems to be no other issue with my heart, not a lot is being done for it. I can get dizzy with it and that horrible thump, thump, thump even when sitting down is now a familiar and unwelcome feeling. Scientists in Canada have mooted the idea that tachycardia, with the heart beating over 100 beats per minute, is yet another symptom of LC. https://www.ctvnews.ca/health/coronavirus/a-spiking-heart-rate-could-be-a-symptom-of-long-covid-experts-say-1.5800252. The positive thing is that, like the palpitations, it doesn't seem to damage the heart. All I can say is I wish it would slow down a bit!

Taste. Pretty much the same as for smell. My sense of taste vanished the first time I contracted Covid during the gannet like consumption of a Burger King meal. Not a bad thing, some would argue! It has been interesting to see whether the taste would come back sooner than the smell and it seems to be ahead at the moment. It's not fully back but I can taste more than in previous months. It's still quite dangerous from the allergen perspective, in that I can't pick up things as sharply as before and have to have a ready supply of antihistamines wherever I go. "I'm allergic to…" is now an essential phrase in restaurants and has to be learned in languages of countries I plan to visit.

Unlike smell, I haven't had any weird substitutes like "this gravy tastes like mayo" but it's like eating and tasting through a plastic box. I'm aware of the taste but it's like my brain can't fully work out how to give me the full experience. Whenever someone else finds a taste particularly strong (that Sicilian lemon gets them every time!), I find I can taste it, even if it is like tasting from behind a window. A work in progress, you may say.

Temperature. Since the third bout of Covid, I have found that my temperature runs at 0.5 to 1 degree higher than 'normal' all the time, increasing when stressed or tired.

A couple of others in a LC chatroom commented on the same strange phenomenon. It's nothing concerning, just a bit bizarre. One paracetamol and the increase in body temp is swiftly brought down to what now passes for my baseline. It's probably not even worth mentioning here but the fact that there are at least four of us with the same symptom made me think I should include it here.

Things need to Change. To mark the first international Long Covid awareness day on 15 March 2023, the LongCovidSoS group created a short film to try to express in less than two minutes what suffering from LC is like. It's short and intense and well worth a look at https://www.longcovidsos.org/awareness. If it does raise awareness and understanding, then we can all potentially benefit. The title says it all and, in my opinion, that's true of the medical profession and the folk on civvy street. Things do need to change. Attitudes need to change. Understanding needs to change if we're got any hope of making a new life with LC.

Travel. With LC causing so many body wide disturbances, it is almost impossible to get travel insurance because even the 'existing problem' companies aren't happy to cover 'unknown' symptoms or ongoing hospital investigations. Couple that with the lung issues I have and the advice not to fly in case they explode, flying abroad doesn't seem to be on my menu any time soon. Cruises leaving from the UK could well be an option but you need heavy travel insurance for that and… see above. Not happening anytime soon.

The UK itself has so much to offer that I'm not viewing my inability to go abroad at the moment as any kind of disaster. Irritating, maybe but not a disaster. However, to go on a staycation, I still have to travel to get there. That's where LC and the fatigue and post exertional malaise kicks in. If I drive, I'm wiped out for two days afterwards, taking out the first two days of a holiday. If I'm a passenger, I'm wiped out for two days afterwards as well. And I have to come home again, meaning that I need to leave at least two days after the return as crash days. Once, it took 10 days to get over a five day break. My options to avoid this seem to be either to spend longer away on holiday or to not go at all. The former adds way too much expense to be practical and the latter is just downright depressing. So at the moment, travelwise, I am a bit stuck! Another reason for the guilt and frustration to come crawling back to haunt me.

Trials. Not as in the trials faced every day by anyone with LC but as in clinical trials that study Long Covid or particular aspects of it. There are a lot out there so it's important to check that it's a legitimate trial before committing to anything. LC is so new that there's no hope of a cure until it's been studied and all aspects are known and identifiable. The only real way forward is to use human guinea pigs. Just like vaccination, it's no one's business other than your own whether you take part in a trial or not and certainly there should be no guilting people with LC into participating in clinical studies or into avoiding them.

I have found some that I would not want to participate in and some that I would. I have done 2 clinical trials so far because I wanted to, not because I felt obliged to. For one, I was in the watch and wait group (i.e. no intervention, just daily diaries) and for the other, I was in the active arm, where I had the treatments. I was made to feel that my contributions were valuable and I was valued as a person. Whatever the outcomes, it's a good feeling to have been involved. But I would never advocate going into something that makes you feel uncomfortable or that you just don't want to do. A fellow LCer commented that his experience with clinical trials was 'brutal' because he was hospitalised with Covid-19 in the pre vaccine days and became part of a trial. When the randomising computer selected him to be part of the no new intervention arm, he felt crushed because his hope of trying one of the experiments for cure or at least help was gone. Of course, he was given proper treatment in the hospital but was left feeling deprived and desolated that a potential cure or help had been denied him by a computer.

If you find a trial that interests you, chat it over with the researchers - they won't mind! Just keep in mind to check for legitimate trials, not something that's not backed properly, has a dodgy sounding set of miracle drugs to try or has no clinical setting.

Tributes.

Always missed
DEARLY
LOVED
FOREVER
IN OUR
HEARTS
ALWAYS
IN OUR
THOUGHTS
LOVED
DEARLY
LOVE
ETERNAL
WE MISS
YOU
EVERYDAY
WE WILL
ALWAYS
REMEMBER
ETERNAL
LOVE
Automatic door
Keep clear
Automatic door
Keep clear

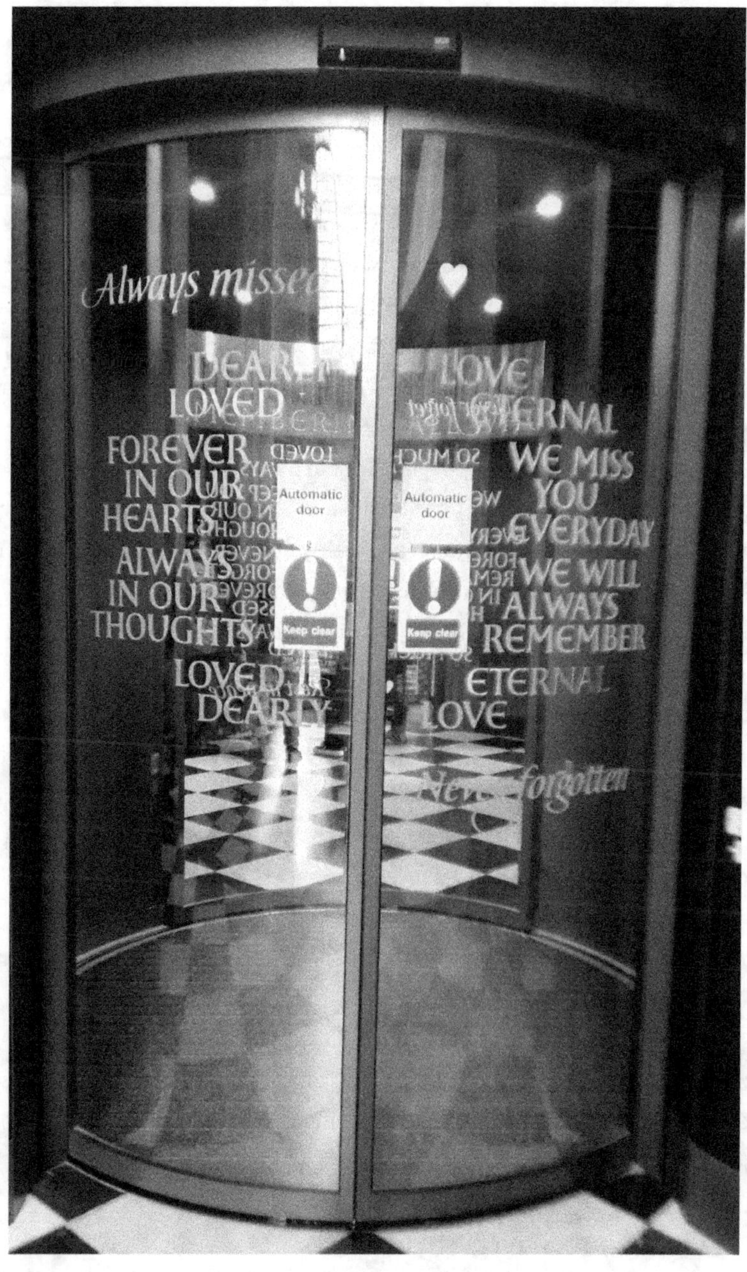

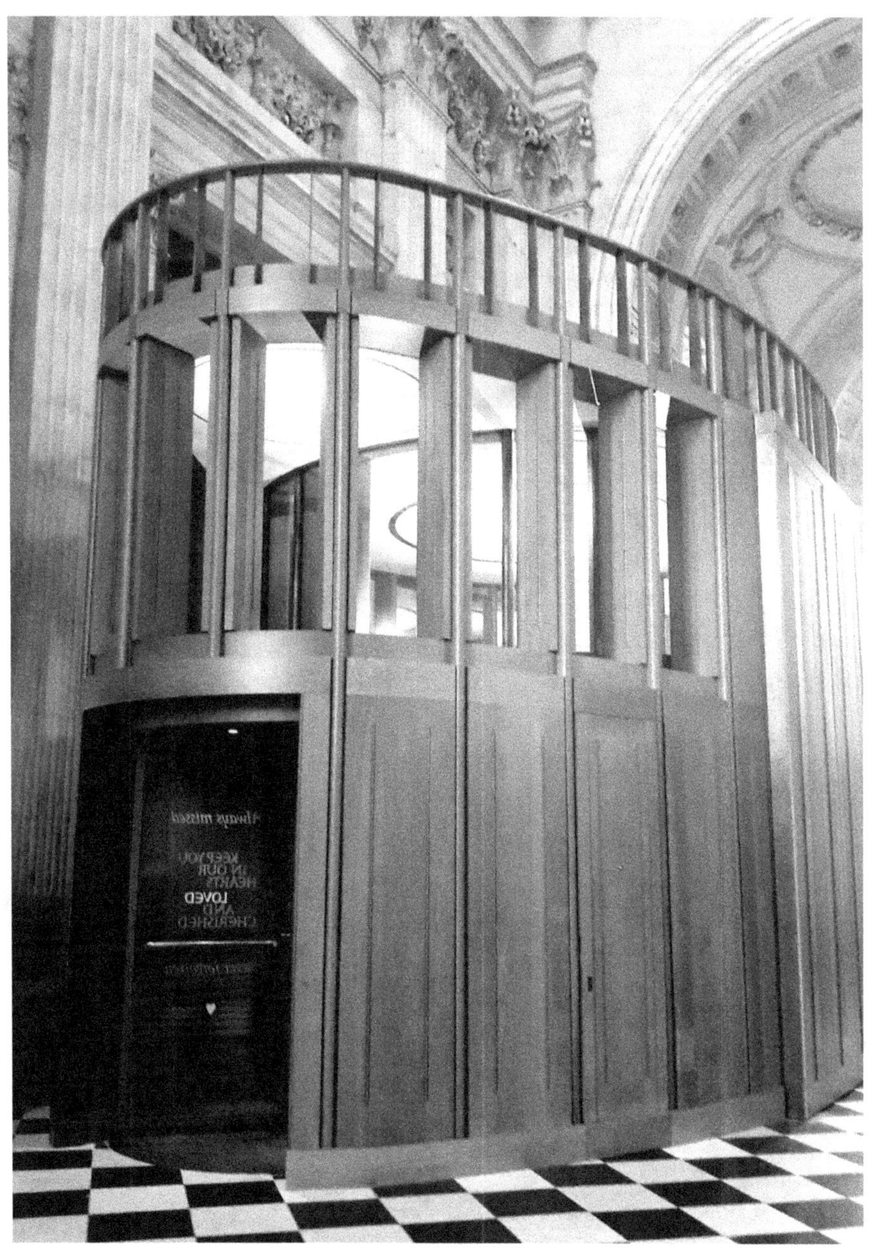

Tribute to those lost to Covid-19 at St Paul's Cathedral, London

It's both heartwarming and hopeful to see that tributes to those lost to Covid-19 are starting to appear. It's important that no one who lost their lives in the pandemic and afterwards is forgotten. Tributes are good for those they left behind. In my dedication at the beginning of the book, I mentioned that those lost to Long Covid are made up of greater numbers than those who died. I mean absolutely no disrespect to the departed or their loved ones and friends by that statement. I want to highlight that death is not the only entity causing people to be lost to Covid.

Weekly, we clapped for the NHS during the height of the pandemic. Every Thursday evening, we stood on our front door steps and clapped, rang bells, pounded saucepans and so on to show our appreciation to all the NHS frontline staff who were literally putting their lives on the line to save us. In 2023, how many of those staff have we lost due to burn out, to being overwhelmed by the relentless charge of Covid, to nervous breakdowns brought on by the pressures of dealing with patients day in, day out, to the constant uncertainty of what the future will bring personally and professionally? They may not have lost their physical lives but we have lost them from the medical profession, some becoming shadows of their former selves.

Taking LC as the topic for this book, most LCers have been lost to Covid too. Psychologists address groups of LCers stating, "The person you used to be is no more, start loving the person you are now." Everything points to a rebirth forced by Covid infection, with physical, mental and emotional changes so uncompromising that it feels the origins of oneself have been lost forever. Research continues and it may be that the whole effect can be reversed but for now, those with LC were also lost to Covid.

I take pictures of tributes to those lost to Covid whenever I see them because I feel it's important for me personally to do so and to see above the parapet of LC. It shows that people care. It proves at some level that LC exists with its inescapable relationship to Covid and the pandemic. There are so many kinds of loss to Covid, still ongoing on a daily basis and it's good to see that tributes are out there and the losses and suffering are recognised.

<u>U is for...</u>

Understanding. There are two branches of understanding that particularly affect me. The first is the obvious one - the understanding of my situation with LC by other people. My emotional day improves drastically every time when someone shows a bit of understanding about LC. I'm not in pain on purpose; I'm not crashing and having to sleep or rest on purpose; I'm not developing new symptoms and trying to work out whether it's LC and ignorable or something serious on purpose. And it's wonderful when someone understands that and either doesn't hassle me because of it or is actually supportive and actively tries to help.

The second kind of definition of understanding is more personal. How there are times and even days where I don't understand much. I don't mean not understanding a specific thing that learning can overcome. I mean having no clue what someone is saying halfway through a conversation, reading a book that suddenly has a load of words strung together and I don't understand what they mean, suddenly not understanding a conversation around me. It's the brain fog of LC that just suddenly wipes out any form of comprehension from my mind until, exactly like with the feelings of being overwhelmed, I have stopped whatever it is and gone away for a 'reset' by sleep, gazing at a wall etc. It strikes at random. There are no obvious triggers apart from it being a guaranteed partner of the LC fatigue, so I can't pre-warn others or get myself into a place of mental (and sometimes physical) safety. I have no idea how to solve this one but have to keep hoping for the support and understanding of others while I do what I can in the moment.

Unlucky dip. LC seems to be an unlucky dip of which symptoms you will develop. They are so wide and so varied that you're never sure whether you have developed a new medical issue or whether it's just another LC trick. And the unlucky dip continues. It doesn't just pick two or three problems and stick with them. No, no. It will pick two or three, add a couple more, delete a couple of the initial ones, add another one or two, re-add one of the deleted ones and so on and so on, making you look like a clueless ignoramus to the medics out there.

Going to the GP with your latest winnings from the unlucky dip can be interesting. I know I have gone in and started with, "I'm sorry to add another thing to my list but…" More tests that prove inconclusive or negative but the symptoms continue. Talking to other LC sufferers is always fascinating because, although we may have different symptoms, there's always a point where the discussion becomes, "Oh you get that too?" "Yes, and do you find that…?" Despite the wild disparity in cases, it seems that some of the products of symptoms, if not the symptoms themselves, have a commonality that LC sufferers can easily identify in one another.

There's no way of avoiding the unlucky dip or predicting when you will be entered again for another prize. It's best to get new symptoms checked out with a long-suffering but amenable GP because, just occasionally, it may not be LC and may be a health condition that can be dealt with because there is information, tested courses of treatment and so on. It's easy to write off new problems to another draw from the LC tombola bucket but, because LC sufferers' health is in constant flux, it's always worth a follow up.

Urgency. There's no doubt about it. Since developing LC, my sense of urgency has changed in two ways. I was always organised and met deadlines, pushing hard to make sure everything that needed to be achieved was achieved at the right time. Brain fog and fatigue put paid to that and I was struggling with even getting out of bed, let alone remembering what I had to do and getting it done in time. This was where my decisions upon what is urgent and what is not came into play. You could call it prioritising but I don't feel it's that organised.

Because my memory is horrible right now, as soon as I get a bill in the post, on email etc, I pay it. No more waiting for payday or until finances dictate it's possible. I don't have that luxury any more. I forget something the second I put it down and unpaid bills are not the way to a harmonious family life! Bills are at the top of my urgent list. See it, pay it, sorted, to misquote a popular UK rail network phrase. It's calming in a way because it's something I can get done and do it right. A new urgency for an everyday occurrence but it works.

Sliding down the urgency scale are big tasks. They get a bit overwhelming, enter into the 'I can't do it' status and never get done, increasing my stress levels as a result, so I become more overwhelmed, meaning less gets done and so on in an ouroboros style loop. I've found an answer with the trusty notepad and pen. Make a list of everything that 'needs' to be done but not in an overarching term. As an example, 'clean the bathroom' now reads 'clean the toilet, clean the sink, clean the bath, clean the floor, clean the tiles' and by just attempting one at a time, the 'I've got to get it done' panic subsides because I can see it is being done, just not at the screeching urgent pace previously demanded.

Urgency has shifted in my mind so that it's less pressure overall, which has led to a calmer outlook on what can and cannot be done and, in a way, has brought more acceptance of my LC limitations. By shifting the urgency goal posts to focus on what is genuinely 100% urgent and what could be done piecemeal over a period of hours, days, weeks etc, the stress has reduced too.

Unpredictability. A theme throughout every symptom of and thought about LC is how unpredictable it is. Patterns prove there is some predictability but, for the most part, LC crashes can strike with no warning. A quiet day, well paced with full rest and calm should lead to a good day the following day, right? Not even 50% of the time! New symptoms can appear without warning and strike at any time. Just the other day, I was walking upstairs, turned to answer a question and, on turning back to continue upwards, completely forgot how to walk upstairs. I was standing a few steps from the top, gazing at the floor, knowing where I wanted to go but just having no clue how to make my body move to get there. I have been climbing stairs for over 50 years but suddenly had to get someone to tell me how to do it.

The unpredictability of LC makes it so hard to plan properly. Even following all the advice on pacing, planning and so on doesn't help sometimes because anything can happen at any given point. The best laid plans are often scuppered due to a sudden, bone crushing fatigue and/or brain fog so bad that I don't even understand what someone is saying to me. What is the answer to this? At the moment, there isn't one other than to be prepared to cancel everything at the last minute, let people down and deal with the inevitable guilt and frustration, all the while hoping that the real LC crashes can be managed enough to be gradually reducing in number and duration. LC's unpredictability leaves this as yet another open question that has no answer.

<u>V is for...</u>

Vaccination. There are Covid vaccines out there and it's not my place to tell anyone to get vaccinated or to refuse vaccination. I caught Covid after my first two vaccinations. I caught it again after my third. And again after my fourth. There's a school of thought that says it would have been a lot worse if I hadn't had the vaccine and another school of thought that says it would have been better if I had avoided vaccination altogether. Personally, I feel I will never know whether it would have been better, worse or exactly the same if I hadn't had the vaccine. If it saved my life, I am very grateful. If it made no difference, so be it. If I would have been better without it, then I have to live with my decision to get vaccinated. I can do that. It's the Long Covid cure vaccine I'm waiting for!

Vision. I hadn't really given a lot of thought to the fact that sometimes my vision was so blurred that even my glasses made no difference, while at others, I almost didn't need my glasses to see quite clearly. I assumed it was part of the ageing process and general eye changes that occur naturally. Then I spoke to a fellow LCer who had experienced the exact same symptoms over a year beforehand. Is it a coincidence or does LC affect vision as well? I can't say because I'm not qualified to do so but, in my opinion, given the changes - temporary or permanent - to other senses such as smell and taste, it doesn't seem a huge stretch to think that vision can be altered too.

I have days where everything is a blur and, because my blood pressure is now controlled by pills and the optician can't find anything wrong/different with my eyes, I have to put it down to another change made by LC to my physiology or brain. The brain MRI didn't show any significant changes in that area but the word significant is noteworthy in itself. What does a neurologist consider significant compared to what is occurring in my body? Is there something showing up but it's obviously (to him) a temporary blip? Or is there just nothing showing, like the blood tests, X rays and so on. Back to sneaky old LC. For what it's worth, I believe LC can affect rather than change vision and I'm hoping it stops playing about with my eyes soon!

Vitamins. It's always worth checking with the GP before starting any fitness or diet regime and that includes using supplements like multi vitamins etc.   Research has shown that people with dysautonomia (autonomic nervous system disorders) can have lower levels of Vitamins D and B12. That includes LCers. Never assume that is your case and get a blood test from the GP to find out. I can't stress that enough and highlight that too much of a good - or unnecessary - thing can be just as harmful as none.

I repeatedly test low for vitamin D, despite taking multi vitamins containing D3 and the GP currently has me on a 4000 iu daily dose to supplement my intake. In theory, it's to help with the fatigue. It doesn't because my fatigue isn't vitamin D based but I take the dose in case it is helping to reset my nervous system. My diet is horrible, although I am trying to make changes, and I have found the difference in general health that taking multi vitamins and an extra dose (GP guided) of Vitamin D3 has made. It may be imperceptible to a blood test or to others but I can feel the difference and it's now part of my morning ritual.

Supplements are a personal choice and should be carefully considered and discussed with a medic before embarking on the superfast mega improvement brands. Lower doses are available and don't seem to be as shocking to the body as the high powered ones. I have found the ones that seem to help me and if I take a few weeks off from taking them, I find my LC symptoms get worse. That could be entirely psychological of course and I would accept that as an explanation. But for now, a lower dose daily seems to be helping me get through every day with LC.

<u>W is for...</u>

Weight loss. This is literally a big part of Covid and LC. With Covid more likely to damage the overweight and LC to make it worse, weight loss seems a bit of a no-brainer in terms of things to do to help yourself. Anyone who hasn't struggled to lose weight will come out with the usual, "Well, eat less, exercise more and lose weight. It's easy, you're just not trying." If it was that easy, I would not have become as obese as I am and stayed that way and nor, I am sure, would many others. I agree that weight loss is an essential ingredient in feeling better because there's not such a strain on the organs and, if combined with exercise, the body can fight off infections fitter because it is quicker. And I am trying to lose that weight and get fit. Thereby hangs the difficulty.

Fatigue absolutely crushes even the best intended weight loss/exercise program. Lowering the carb intake leads to - wait for it - fatigue and sugar cravings. Unaccustomed exercise leads to - again - fatigue. The problems I'm having, even with an NHS recommended weight loss plan, is that by trying to follow all the guidelines, recipes and exercise suggestions, I am getting more and more fatigued. As yet, there has been no specific LC designed weight loss and exercise program, so again one size does not fit all. It wouldn't even fit all the LCers who want to lose weight because we all have such a variety of symptoms and everything standard just worsens a lot of symptoms.

That doesn't mean I don't try. I am following, as close as my LC allows, an NHS guided programme. By having few or no carbs in my evening meal, I have noticed that the inflammation in my joints has improved. It's still there but it has improved. That can only be a good thing. One week, I lose a couple of pounds but the fatigue hits so I regain them the following week. It's a case of swings and roundabouts so I am focussing not so much on the weight loss but trying to eat smarter and healthier and hoping that benefits like less joint pain flare ups become more and more regular. Maybe once that happens, I can focus on weight loss itself. Who knows, a healthier eating pattern may result in some natural weight loss without a lot of effort on my part. It's part of the plan for the future that I am trying to work towards now.

Who am I? It's a question I keep asking myself because I don't know who I am any more. I'm certainly not who I used to be, thanks to all the changes forced on me by LC. Some changes, I have to admit to quite liking, while others cause me a lot of anguish and hours awake ruminating over. I'm not going to list over another 100 pages every change I feel has happened to me so I will share a positive and a negative and move on. Was that a cry of 'Thank the Lord for that!' I just felt rippling through the ether?!

Some positives may not seem to be such to an outsider and so it may not be instantly understandable why I like being less of a dogsbody and having a far lower tolerance for those around me treating me and speaking to me like I am a naughty child. My intolerance for people acting like idiots has hit rock bottom, along with my patience. I just don't have the physical, emotional or mental capacity any more for pushing it down inside myself, grimacing and saying nothing. I can't say I shout back now because I don't but my sarcasm level has increased exponentially (when I can get the words out!) and, instead of my old habit of trying to make up for my obvious shortcomings and rush to help or sort out the other person's problems, I raise my hands, say 'I can't help you then,' or 'I'm not being a part of this conversation any more,' and move away. It is emotionally draining to do this but actually, the overall burden is easier when I do. LC means I don't have the mental capacity any more to retain it all (everything I have done wrong just goes on longer than *Lord of the Rings*!) and I get way too fatigued to keep going over and over it with whomever is spouting my iniquities at me. That's if I've even managed to decipher what the issue is in the first place! I'm feeling this is a positive step in my life. It is interesting that I begin with a positive rather than a negative example. That's a new me.

I'm not the intelligent being that I once was. That hurts and causes me a lot of mental anguish. I loved learning, solving problems, discovering new things and mentally exploring. I try every day with the brain training games and apps but I'm still not able to piece information together properly or put it into a reasonable frame any more and get distracted faster than a goldfish with the overall comprehensive ability of an amoeba . The worst part about it is that I am aware of it and every daily failure hurts. The other day, I helped my daughter compose a letter of complaint. Pre LC, I could have done that, not needed to check it and posted it within an hour. This took the best part of four hours to write a single page, with a lack of words and erudition, followed by constant revisions of grammar and syntax. It frustrates the hell out of me and underlines daily that I'm not who I used to be. This is one of the biggest negatives for the new version of me.

Who am I now? That might be a better way of phrasing it than who am I. I feel there's no doubt that LC has changed me physically, mentally and emotionally. I didn't think I'd ever feel positively about exercise and wanting to improve the way I eat but equally I never thought I would forget how to open a door with a push down handle! I think why I feel so aggrieved about it all is that I have had no choice in the vast majority of the changes that have happened. I could go on and on giving examples but I hope that you, as the reader, will take it on trust that these literal life-changing things have happened to me, continue happening and never fail to surprise and/or horrify me. "Who am I now?" is an unanswerable question because it is built on constantly shifting sands.

The changes to self happen, in different ways and at different levels, to every LCer. Some people find the changes small and manageable, some argue they are barely noticeable but they are still there. Others literally have their pre-existing lives ripped away from them, being left with a completely new, scary way of living. When this happens, you are left with the somewhat navel-gazing question of, "Who am I now?" And it's quite hard to answer that question and even more difficult to decide whether you like the new you or not. How to change the things you really don't like is the age old question that so many self-help books have sought to solve over decades. There is no answer to that one, I feel. "Who am I?" can almost be seen as a vigilance thing for LCers and is perhaps not a bad thing to review occasionally.

Words. Words used to flow easily for me, be it verbally or on paper. Now, I find I have to think before almost every word I utter and even then, I am struggling to find a word or phrase. Sometimes, the words just don't come at all, while at other times, I stammer and stammer and eventually they pop out. It's like my brain just erases whole sentences between brain and mouth and no amount of recall attempts can fill in the blanks. It's part of the brain fog but also different to the brain fog. When the brain fog is bad, the terms just don't come, full stop. When the brain fog is okay or manageable, the scary thing is that words still elude me or I say completely the wrong word in place of the right one. "Pass me the melon to cut the cake," was an interesting one.

I don't know if my words will come back, whether it is all part of LC that may improve if my brain rewires itself or whether it is only going to get worse. The LC rehab clinics and neurologists alike are strangely silent on the topic, telling me and my fellow LCers, "Of course it's not dementia, it's just brain fog," without understanding just how scary it is to be losing your ability to communicate clearly with others in a variety of situations. At hospital appointments, it is frustrating and annoying to fail to pass on what you consider to be key information because the words just won't come and it certainly doesn't help with curing the problem.

The other aspect of words that is particularly relevant to me since getting LC is understanding of words. I get to the stage in conversations where I am sitting in a pool of panic because I just don't understand what is being said to me and around me. It's like the brain just suddenly switches off the comprehension button and all that happens is words cascade around me, meaning literally nothing, even though they are spoken in my mother tongue. I can hear just fine but the actual words may as well be in a language I don't speak. Again, in a hospital scenario, that can be very frightening because often I have no idea what I am agreeing to - sometimes it has been a medical procedure, others it has been agreeing to be discharged even when the problem is ongoing. In a social situation, it can look as though I don't want to join in or am sulking because I am sitting there, trying to process the words falling around me and cannot participate in the conversation because I need minutes at a time to try to catch up with what is being said. And when I have caught up, the topic has changed and people have moved on, making any comments from me irrelevant to the current conversation and even a bit bizarre. I am far from alone in this and fellow LCers have told me that they have exactly the same problems in groups or even one to one situations. I find it applies to the written word as well and very often cannot follow a plot in a novel or have to re-read the same paragraph over and over in an instruction manual or hospital letter. The words, if I have understood them, just fade away from me as if I had never read them. Other times, I find reading even children's books (thanks, Enid Blyton!) helps my mind gear up to the day ahead or relax in the evening.

"But she's written over 45,000 words in this book so she's clearly capable of using words so must be exaggerating," are comments I can almost hear non LCers thinking. I don't deny that and all the words here are my own (apart from the quoted and attributed ones). They have taken the best part of a year to write, with the facility for me to look up synonyms, edit and alter time and time again. That's very different to the instant bam bam bam of words in a dialogue or group situation. There's no response required and time lapses don't matter. That's the difference.

Even apps like Words With Friends can be a challenge. On a relatively brain fog free day, I can play quite easily (not necessarily well - I wouldn't claim that!) On a day where my brain is like a very thick jelly, I can manage 2 letter words at best. My loss rate is phenomenal but it makes the occasional win even sweeter, with the hope that every so often, there's a little ray of light making my words shine as they come back to me and I can use them in the game.

As with everything LC, I have no idea if I will ever be able to have a normal conversation again without searching for words or understanding. It is frustrating and upsetting to be like this and see the pity and disdain in others' eyes as I struggle to communicate. Even more hurtful is the rolling hand with the 'get a move on with it' gesture. I can't help it and doing that to me just makes the stress level higher and the words come even slower. I keep using word game apps, IQ tests, DS brain training games and so on to try and trigger some spark in my brain to rewire, to heal so that I can once more speak, understand, read and listen with full comprehension.

Work. There are two aspects to the theme of work that spring instantly to mind. There's the fact that I haven't been in paid employment since I developed LC but also the question of whether employers have to make the 'reasonable adjustments' identified in the UK's 2010 Equality Act because LC is a recognised disability. Quite a large topic that is discussed ad infinitum in other literature but work merits an entry here because it's a big part of life with and without LC.

I can't concentrate long enough (more than 30 minutes at a time on a good day for the whole day) and I get fatigued too fast to be able to hold down a job, even with the most reasonable adjustments in the world being made for me. This leads to difficulties financially but also psychologically because I feel that I now contribute very little to the family and home. It's also a bit of a circle of despair, in that I don't get extra stimulation by working but can't get extra stimulation by working because I can't work, thanks to the effects of LC upon me. It is a very depressing situation to be in, again with the huge guilt factor for the effect it is having on my family, as well as awareness of the burdens placed on them with my incapacity, looming large over the whole thing. It's a bit of a conundrum and I can only hope to keep plugging away, moving the baseline so that one day, I may be employed again and contributing to society and my family.

There raged quite a debate on whether or not LC is a disability and whether employers had to make allowances for LCers. There is always the inevitable and unenviable task of weeding out the lead-swingers, the exaggerators and the plain idle from the genuine cases and I don't envy employers that job. However, once veracity has been proven as much as it ever can be, the question arises of whether a place of employment should make reasonable adjustments for an LCer. It's intangible, it's unpredictable and it's too new to be one of the 'official disabilities'.

The answer came following an employment tribunal in Scotland. The full details of the judgment can be found at https://assets.publishing.service.gov.uk/media/62a1feace90e07039e31b82c/Mr_T_B urke_v_Turning_Point_Scotland_-_4112457.2021_-_Preliminary.pdf Essentially, Terence Burke claimed disability discrimination and unfair dismissal after his sacking by Turning Point, Scotland, because of his LC. The tribunal upheld Mr Burke's claims and gave him permission to pursue his claim for disability discrimination, as his LC symptoms met the relevant criteria to be classed as a disability. Employers now have no excuse for wriggling on the 'reasonable adjustments' line and many LCers I have spoken to have commented very positively on their bosses' willingness to comply. Not all, obviously, but it's a hell of a start.

Whilst that is excellent news, it's a real minefield for the self-employed. If you don't work, you don't get paid, which is my current problem. A psychologist in an LC clinic even went as far as to tell a fellow self-employed LCer to work less and it would reduce his fatigue and brain fog. And is this 'genius' psychologist offering to make up the financial shortfall? Absolutely not. This brings in the knotty problem of benefits and eligibility. Essentially, after having LC for 12 months, we have the potential to be classed as disabled and claim Personal Independence Payments. All well and good but currently that is less than £70 a week for the standard rate. Not enough for a family to live on and there's also the issue of people not wanting to be on benefits because they would rather work.

The biggest slap in the face is being ineligible to get help or advice with getting paid employment (or self employed work) because you're not on benefits due to your savings being too large to get help until you've used them up and are on benefits. It's a ridiculous merry-go-round that those with disabilities have known for a long time. To get help with employment, you have to use any savings over the bench-mark, go on to benefits and then get advice and help. I'm not advocating that folk with huge amounts stashed in banks and offshore accounts should be paid benefits, not at all. But what if all that's needed, especially for those with disabilities, is some advice, guidance and perhaps an introduction to an appropriate, sympathetic employer? Surely it's counter-productive to refuse that and cost the tax-payers more money after the savings have gone because, due to lack of facilitation, benefits are the only remaining choice. That's if the benefits are even approved. When I argue that, even if it was only one morning a month, people whose savings are too large for eligibility could drop in to a Job Centre for advice and guidance to completely avoid going on to benefits, get a suitable job and thereby save the tax-payer a lot of money, I'm met with a blank stare and, "That's not how the system works." It's an odd, self-defeating system, in my opinion, that LCers are going to have to learn to navigate.

<u>X is for...</u>

X-Rays. A bit predictable for the letter X but actually quite interesting too. I was recently admitted to hospital with Influenza A and had some chest X-Rays to see how wide spread my problem was. The doctors compared it to previous X-Rays, which had been taken before and after LC came to stay. What was interesting was the appearance of patches (a technical term?!) in my left lung following the second Covid infection, which increased slightly with the Influenza A infection. The doctor wasn't too forthcoming on the question of whether these patches were permanent or not, probably because they just don't know yet, or whether my lung is permanently damaged.

Too often, traditional X-Rays are discarded in favour of the MRI route but I wonder if they could have a vital part to play in the study of LC. If looking at 3 X-Rays taken over a period of 3 years can show that Covid damaged my lung and it has not healed, only to be further affected by more traditional infections like Influenza, then who knows what information a series of X-Rays over a shorter period of time in a variety of LC individuals could yield? Cheaper and more accessible for the NHS and 100% more inclusive for those of us too terrified of MRIs to be able to participate in any treatments or research studies, I'd ask someone in the medical profession to give the humble X-Ray a thought when proposing a new LC study.

Xenon. A gas that behaves in a similar way to oxygen that, when hyperpolarised and viewed in an MRI scanner, can show whether there have been lung changes in those with LC. Ordinary scans - CT or MRI - don't show any changes. Xenon was used in an initial study by Explain (and will be used in a larger study) to look at the gas transfer from the lungs to the bloodstream in LC sufferers. Unsurprisingly to those of us with LC, the gas transfer is impaired by damage to the lungs caused by Covid but all the patients involved in the study had already had normal results from X-rays, CT scans and MRIs without the Xenon gas. Again, this demonstrates my thinking that the markers are there for LC but there are no standardised

markers/clues identified for diagnosticians to look for. Yet. Keep watching for the
Xenon studies - they could be our only hope of proof.

<u>Y is for...</u>

Yeah, I get it. The words that many people with a long term diagnosis or a disability get huge relief from hearing. It can only come from someone who has the same diagnosis because, much as medics and family and friends want to understand, no one can unless they are in exactly the same boat. That's not a criticism, it's a fact. For me, it's a relief from the prison of my thoughts to hear someone say, "Yeah, I get it," when I'm talking with them about a shared aspect of LC. Someone else understands. Someone else identifies. It's great to be able to talk about shared experiences but, for me, it's even better to know that someone else can identify with the sometimes indescribable things in my head about what I'm going through. I'm not going mad; I'm not just making stuff up; the pain is real; the thoughts I have are not unusual. Someone else truly gets it. It's a catharsis of sorts and strangely relaxing too.

Year. January 2023 saw the media incorrectly trumpeting the results of a study published in the BMJ where, amongst other things, the authors of the paper hypothesised that LC goes away naturally after a year, stating *"patients with mild covid-19 are at risk for a small number of health outcomes, most of which are resolved within a year from diagnosis"*. (https://www.bmj.com/content/380/bmj-2022-072529) This led to many of my friends and involved medical professionals telling me that LC would soon be over and my life would be back to normal. When I commented that I was already 17 months into my LC life, along with many fellow LCers who were 2+ years into the journey, they fell silent and looked puzzled. "But I read that…" became a very familiar phrase.

What the initial media hype failed to notice was that the BMJ published a rapid response to this article on the same day. In it, Jeremy Rossman et al point out that *"the study likely presents an overly optimistic view of Long Covid recovery."* (https://www.bmj.com/content/380/bmj-2022-072529/rr-1) This response gave a clearer picture of what LC is like but the media ignored it in favour of the big headlines about cures, recovery and so on, which actually set me and fellow LCers back a lot both socially and medically and definitely in terms of understanding.

Some people do recover within a year and there has been talk that it has been those with the Covid-19 Omicron infection who have made up a large percentage of those. I can't comment on the veracity or otherwise of this but the LCers I have dealings with mainly come from the original, Alpha and Delta infections and have all had LC for at least 18 months, many now passing for their 3 year anniversary. Although I do know of someone with the original strain who had been hospitalised who no longer has LC. My point is that although in some cases it does, LC doesn't clear up after a year for huge numbers of LCers like myself. The media isn't always the font of knowledge and can get it very wrong.

For LCers, the knock on effect of this 'Long Covid goes away after a year' thinking is that it is now harder to get new help medically, with benefits, at work and socially because we've had it too long and the papers say we are cured so we must be swinging the lead. The element of disbelief that exists for all invisible illnesses has grown again because of this one study's results being splashed across all media platforms. In short, LC lasts longer than a year for many people, regardless of what the papers say. I would love to be able to have an end point for my LC - ooh, only another 20 days to go - but the question of permanence remains. It could be with some of us for the rest of our lives, as we may not be around long enough to see a cure or effective management. A year is optimistic and also crushing when you are 3+ years in!

<u>Z is for...</u>

Zombie days. Not the same as a duvet day, when all you want to do is snuggle down in bed. Zombie days are when you can't understand what people are saying to you, can't make yourself understood, can't move, can't think and just generally exist. It's as if life support has been turned down to minimum power. It's a full on LC crash but not one that goes away after a few hours of rest and isn't necessarily just for a day. It can be for a few days or weeks. I've been lucky because the longest Zombie session I have had lasted 10 days. Some LC folk are looking at weeks and months in a row rather than days here and there.

It affects your ability to plan anything because your health is suddenly unpredictable. The Zombie days are unpredictable, so you can't think, "Oh well, I'm bound to have a Zombie day next Thursday so I'll keep the day free." Zombie days are not the usual fatigue, post exertional malaise etc. They are full out shutdowns that can't be predicted or avoided. Like a lot of the LC symptoms, they just have to be got through. That can be made easier by the understanding of those around you - family, work colleagues, medical professionals. And they can be made even harder when those individuals don't understand, which is a main reason why I decided to create this mini guide to the challenges of Long Covid. To help others understand when you just can't explain it.

Is there an end?

Every so often, I try to almost review myself in a 'who am I now?' way. I try to take anything good and positive that has been forced upon me and like it, making it something to try and nurture. When it's the bad stuff, like the impatience and the intolerance, I try to be aware of it and try to do a little bit of weeding it out when I notice it is happening. If there's some stuff I can't change either for good or bad, I'm trying to accept it. I'm trying (often failing!) to improve my overall nutrition and fitness levels but LC frequently challenges those ambitions. But where does that ultimately leave me?

The open ended nature of LC makes it hard to see an end to it all or light at the end of the tunnel or however you want to express it. It's an acceptance through gritted teeth almost and a need to try to get as good as it gets not as good as it was. Some LCers say they are grateful because LC has brought some positive changes to their thinking, relationships and lifestyle. Good on them. I am genuinely delighted that something positive has come of this for some people.

For me, it's a case of plodding on, trying to improve my LC and improve my acceptance of it and adapt to a radically different mind set as well as physical and mental abilities. It's a case of plodding on with research into LC because no one out there is going to tell you anything - you need to find it out for yourself and then keep nagging the relevant medics about it to try and get some treatment. A lot of LC help is self led because there are no answers out there or they are so well hidden and perhaps too expensive to be shared with the general populace.

It would be lovely to think that, one day, you could rock up to a clinic or a doctor with your LC and say, "Please fix me," and they will. Maybe one day that will happen but for now, keep on plodding. Keep on sharing with family and friends. Keep explaining it to make everyone's life a bit easier, certainly on the understanding front. I hope this collection of thoughts and experiences has helped you to feel not so alone with LC and has also helped those you care about to understand what is going on with your LC and perhaps be more tolerant of it.

To all the LCers out there, you're amazing. Hang in there. Worrying about tomorrow only takes away the peace of today. To all those who read this book to understand what their loved one/friend/patient/colleague is going through, bless you.

Let's hope for a cure and if there's no cure, let's hope for universal understanding, patience and tolerance. Here endeth the lesson.

<u>References and Useful links</u>

Below is a list of links and books that I have either used and quoted here or found online and felt may be of some use. A Google search throws up so many Long Covid references that it's exhausting just scrolling down the page, never mind accessing them. The list below is obviously incomplete but I look on it as a starting point that can lead on to other links, other information and articles that interest you personally. I found them and the books detailed after the weblinks helpful to me. The books have pages and pages of references to scientific papers in their latter pages, which again is a good kicking off point. More and more LC books are being published (like this one!) so I can't claim these are the only or the best books available. They are ones that helped me and I plan to read many more and access more web pages too. It's a never-ending quest to find information, probably that will only cease once a cast iron cure is found. Enjoy this list and enjoy your own searches too. There's a lot of information out there - have fun finding what speaks to you!

https://assets.publishing.service.gov.uk/media/62a1feace90e07039e31b82c/Mr_T_Burke_v_Turning_Point_Scotland_-_4112457.2021_-_Preliminary.pdf

https://www.darksideofsleepingpills.com/

https://hiddendisabilitiesstore.com/uk/long-covid-card.html

https://imperial.ac.uk/medicine/research-and-impact/groups/react-study/studies/react-long-covid/ has a useful poster of LC symptoms to download

https://patientresearchcovid19.com/

https://thedysautonomiaproject.org/lcad/

https://www.bmj.com/content/380/bmj-2022-072529 and the response at
https://www.bmj.com/content/380/bmj-2022-072529/rr-1

https://www.brownejacobson.com/insights/long-covid-and-whether-this-amounts-to-a-disability

https://www.dailymail.co.uk/health/article-11792693/Long-Covid-doubles-chances-life-threatening-heart-problems-study-finds.html

https://www.england.nhs.uk/2020/10/nhs-to-offer-long-covid-help/

https://www.gov.uk/definition-of-disability-under-equality-act-2010#:~:text=You're%20disabled%20under%20the,to%20do%20normal%20daily%20activities.

https://www.gov.uk/guidance/find-help-and-support-if-you-have-long-covid

https://www.longcovidsos.org/awareness for the Things Need to Change short film.

https://www.longcovidsos.org/

https://ncimi.co.uk/latest/xenon-gas-and-mri-scans-show-hidden-lung-damage-in-long-covid-patients/
https://www.nytimes.com/2021/03/17/opinion/long-covid.html

https://www.ridgmountpractice.nhs.uk/pulse-oximeters for the oximeter charts

https://www.thetimes.co.uk/article/loss-of-smell-in-long-covid-patients-caused-by-immune-response-say-scientists-htz0tvldm (George Sandeman article)

https://www.youtube.com/watch?v=gHJSYEITRZQ (for the Dr Boon Lim breathing technique)

Dalton-Smith, Saundra (2018) *Sacred Rest: Recover your Life, Renew your Energy, Restore your Sanity* FaithWords publishers

Gahan, Lucy (2022) *Breaking Free from Long Covid* Jessica Kingsley Publishers

Gardner, David (2022) *Covid 19 The Conspiracy Theories* Jon Blake Publishing Ltd

Medinger, Gez & Altmann, Danny (2022) *The Long Covid Handbook* Penguin Books

Specialists at Post-Covid Clinic, Oxford (2022) *The Long Covid self help guide* Green Tree, Bloomsbury Publishing PLC

Walker, Matthew (2017) *Why We Sleep*, Penguin Books

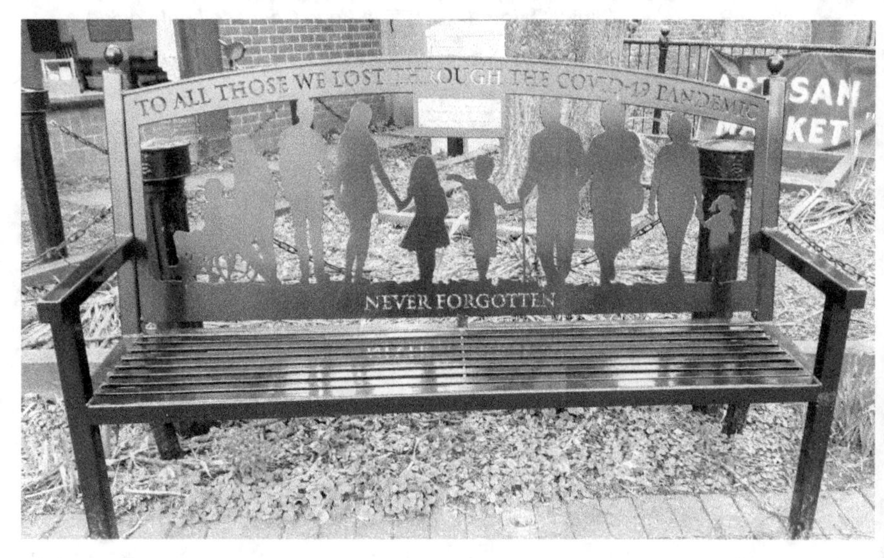

TO ALL THOSE WE LOST THROUGH THE COVID-19 PANDEMIC
NEVER FORGOTTEN
ARTISAN MARKET